Diet and Cancer

Diet and Cancer

An Anthroposophical Contribution to Cancer Prevention

Udo Renzenbrink

Translated by
Johanna Collis and Anna Meuss

Rudolf Steiner Press, London
Raphael Medical Centre, Hildenborough

Translated from the original German: *Diät bei Krebs. Was tun zur Vorsorge?*
published by 'Arbeitskreis für Ernährungsforschung e.V.', D-7263 Bad Liebenzell-
Unterlengenhardt, 1982.

ISBN 0-85440-766-9

Typeset by Grassroots, London N3 2LJ
Printed in Great Britain

CONTENTS

Introduction

1   The Nature of Man. What is a Carcinoma?
The Components of Man's Being 1

2   Do Some Foods Produce Tumour Growth by
Overburdening the Body's Metabolism? The
Importance of the Vitality of Foods 6

3   Cancer-Causing Foreign Substances in
Environment and Food 10

4   Disorders of the Fluid Organism. Abnormal
Etheric Growth Forces Generate Cell
Proliferation. Tomatoes, Potatoes,
Fungi (Mushrooms), Meat 14

5   The Cancer Cell Fails to Breathe.
Respiratory Function and Nutrition 20

6   Disorders of Light Metabolism in Cancer
Patients. The Light Quality of Foods 25

7   The Cancer Cell as a Cold Focus. Stimulating
the Warmth Organism by Nutrition 29

8   Silica Processes which Provide Form. Filling
the Form with Light and Warmth 33

9   The Liver as the Chief Organ for Metabolism
and Detoxification. The Liver and Cancer.
Diet as a Preventative Measure 36

10   Rhythms 40

11   Cereal Grains in the Diet of Cancer Patients 48

12   Practical Guidelines 51

Cultivation and processing of Plant Products
Cereal Grains
Herbs and Spices
Milk and Dairy Products
Vegetables
Lactic-fermented Produce
Fruits
Fats
Sugar
Honey
Meat
Beverages
High Fibre Diet
Raw Food Diet
Breuss's Vegetable Juice Cure
The Importance of Regular Mealtimes
Suggested Daily Menu

Conclusion 62

Bibliography and Addresses 63

INTRODUCTION

In industrialized countries every fourth death is caused by cancer. Scarcely any family or circle of acquaintance is spared the sad fate of watching while a loved one slowly succumbs to this illness. Those who have faced the knowledge that their body is carrying a tumour which is threatening to spread may well ask: What can I expect from the future? Must I give in without a fight or are there practical and promising methods for tackling the situation?

The growth of a tumour is usually preceded by years of non-specific disorders in various parts of the metabolism, so that the tumour itself is only the final stage of the process. But these preliminary conditions do not always inevitably lead to the growth of a tumour. They can be controlled by the organism, can remain static, or life may simply not be long enough for a growth to develop.

The tendency to tumour formation is widespread. Those who use capillary dynamolysis or Pfeiffer's copper-chloride crystallization method to analyse blood are alarmed by the signs of a predisposition to cancer in almost every sample they test. All sections of the population are in need of overall measures with which to combat this disposition to cancer.

An approach in which nutrition is used to prevent the development of cancer can justifiably be termed 'prophylactic'. This is a term wrongly used by health authorities today to mean no more than the early discovery of a tumour, yet this has nothing to do with prevention as such.

It is the purpose of this book to discuss nutrition as a means of preventing cancer. Our concern is not with complicated rules to which it is difficult to adhere but with a wholefood diet that is in harmony with the total human being. However, because of the seriousness and prevalence of cancer today, a degree of consistency and determination is necessary both in avoiding certain products and in attending to quality in the composition and preparation of food.

Cancer is as many-sided and varied as human beings and their evolution. This is why, despite colossal efforts, scientific medicine has reached few insights into the causes and nature of this disease. Its customary treatment by means of operation, radiation and chemotherapy is concerned only with the tumour itself, and takes no account of factors which underlie the illness as a whole.

On the basis of Rudolf Steiner's Anthroposophy, our point of departure will be a holistic approach to the human being who may be seen as possessing not only a physical body but also an etheric body, an astral body and the ego. It will be seen that every aspect of the human being is affected by cancer and that this finds differing expression in the various parts. Taking the many-sided nature of cancer into account in this way, it is possible to discover guidelines for suitable dietary measures.

Frequent references to Rudolf Steiner's suggestions and direct quotations from his lectures and books make clear which of our statements are based on findings he arrived at through his method of spiritual research. This method has pushed back the limits of science and brought into consideration reliable knowledge from the realm of the spirit. His book *Knowledge of the Higher Worlds* describes the system of exercises which makes this method accessible to anyone who might be interested.

1. THE NATURE OF MAN
WHAT IS A CARCINOMA?

The Components of Man's Being

The *physical body* is the only visible part of the human being, consisting as it does of the substances which also go to make up the external world. But its form and the way it functions cannot be fully explained in the mechanistic and causal terms used to describe inanimate mineral substances. Whatever we observe about the human organism, every form and every process is comprehensible only when seen as an expression of spirit and soul. Man's upright stance, the way an individual moves and walks, each person's manner of speaking, the way people look on the world, but also the way they think, feel and act—none of this arises from the physical body, for it is all an expression of the way spirit and soul work within the body. All these processes involve every part of the organism, even the finest cell structures and their functions. The physical body was created out of the deepest wisdom in order to serve as a tool for spirit and soul.

This physical body is maintained by creative forces, for left to itself it would disintegrate, as does a corpse, in accordance with the laws of the mineral world. This logical conclusion alone is sufficient basis on which to accept that these creative forces do exist. Over and above this, it is possible to achieve, through appropriate exercises, a view of this world of creative forces as a supersensible system of forces which transcends what the senses of the physical body can behold. Though physical eyes cannot see it, we call it the etheric body or life body because in its whole configuration and arrangement it resembles a body.

Plants as well as human beings possess an *etheric body*. It is the bearer of growth and procreation; it stimulates and guides metabolism, and it is the vehicle for the principle which gives form to the physical body. The heaviness of the physical body's solid substances is overcome in a way which enables them to be taken up by a higher order, namely that of the creative forces. Thus another name for the etheric

1

body is the 'body of creative forces'. While the mineral element is expressed in the physical body, the etheric creative forces weave in the fluid element. There is no life without water.

The third component of man's being, the *astral body*, also called the 'sentient body', is the bearer of pain and joy, of drives and emotions. The name refers to its connection with the world of the stars; it is a 'star body'. Plants possess only a physical and an etheric body, but animals as well as human beings have an astral body. Just as the etheric body comes to realization in the rhythmical movements of the fluid element, so is the astral body linked to the organism via the element of air, the stream of the breath.

Among all created things of the earth, human beings alone possess an *ego*. Creatures who are able to call themselves 'I' bear within them a world of their own which can be comprehended by thinking. Something spiritual speaks in them, something towards which the ego can learn to feel responsible and indebted. The voice of conscience stirs. The ego, too, creates its own organization in the body, something which enables it, far beneath the threshold of consciousness, to shape functions and structures in the body in a way which befits not only human beings in general but also the individual in particular. No human organism is identical with any other. Brow, countenance, hands, indeed the total human form, are expressions of a unique, unmistakable personality. This individual stamp reaches right down to the physical substances of the body. For instance, there are as many forms of protein as there are or ever were human beings on the earth. The element of warmth opens up the material world for the ego, and its organic basis is the blood. It was not for nothing that Mephistopheles required Faust to sign with his own blood. It is an expression of man's eternal entelechy.

The Four Components of the Human Being

Human Being	Realms of Nature	Elements
physical body	mineral	earth
etheric body	plant	water
astral body	animal	air
ego	man	fire

The Threefold Human Being

The anthroposophical view of man takes account not only of the four components—ego, astral body, etheric body, physical body—but also of the human organism in its threefold aspect. Thus a distinction is made between the system of nerves and senses centred in the head, the rhythmical system represented by heart and lungs, and the system of metabolism and limbs.

These three spheres are the source of activities which enliven and maintain the total organism. In them live the invisible components of man's being, etheric body, astral body and ego. But the way they relate to the three spheres of the physical organism differs.

The system of nerves and senses. In the sense organs, the ego, the astral body and to some extent the etheric body are only loosely connected with the physical body. As a sense organ evolved, these aspects partially withdrew from its organic formation and began to serve the actual activity of perception, which is a living process that takes place in the soul. The eye may serve as an example. In it the physical body is to quite an extent self-sufficient. The eye can be almost entirely explained in accordance with physical laws for it is, as Rudolf Steiner put it, 'nature's camera'. In the eye, the etheric body is largely free of the physical body and is thus able—in the activity of sense perception—to unite with whatever lies outside the body. The situation is similar with regard to the ear.

In the brain and in the nerves, too, etheric creative powers are freed and thus enabled to serve the 'higher' components, namely astral body and ego, in the structuring of processes of spirit and soul.

The rhythmic system. Here the etheric body does not turn outwards, as in the senses, but remains bound up with the physical body, filling it with life with the help of the fluid organism. Ego and astral body work rhythmically in the physical body. In every in-drawn breath they permeate it, and then they withdraw again. The beat of the pulse is oriented to this sequence of functions. The astral body uses the element of air for its activity.

The Threefold Human Organism

1. *System of Nerves and Senses*

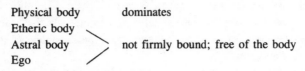

    Physical body   dominates
    Etheric body
    Astral body   not firmly bound; free of the body
    Ego

2. *Rhythmic System*

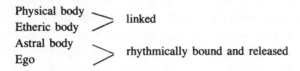

    Physical body   linked
    Etheric body
    Astral body   rhythmically bound and released
    Ego

3. *System of Metabolism and Limbs*

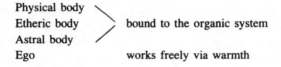

    Physical body
    Etheric body   bound to the organic system
    Astral body
    Ego   works freely via warmth

The system of metabolism and limbs. In metabolism, the astral body as well as the etheric body is bound to the physical body. The activity of the astral body consists in creating inner space in different ways in the various organs.

In metabolism, the ego gives form to the physical processes far beneath the threshold of consciousness. And the ego approaches the limbs by means of movement, to which it gives its individual stamp. Thus the manner in which people move is most revealing with regard to the character of their ego. Here it is the element of warmth that provides the link for the ego with the physical body.

Tumours grow when the components of the human being are prevented from working into the various parts of the organism. This will be discussed in later chapters as shown in the following summary.[1,2]

4

Development and Healing of Cancer in Relation to the Components of Man's Being

Mineral body **Physical body**	Burdened by 'dead' foodstuffs; methods of cultivation; devitalisation; additives	Chapters 2 and 3
Fluid organism **Etheric body**	Disorders of protein and fat metabolism; distorted etheric growth forces	Chapter 4
Air organism **Astral body**	Cell respiration; pathological fermentation; significance of added respiratory enzymes and lactic-fermented products; sugar	Chapter 5
Light organism **Astral Body**	Failure of cancer cells to radiate light; light quality of foodstuffs	Chapter 6
Warmth organism **Ego**	The cancer cell as a cold focus; the warmth quality of foodstuffs	Chapter 7

2. DO SOME FOODS PROMOTE TUMOUR GROWTH BY OVERBURDENING THE BODY'S METABOLISM?

The Importance of the Vitality of Foods

Tumours form when the play of forces between the etheric and the physical body is disturbed. Rudolf Steiner describes[3] how the physical body absorbs too strongly the forces from its environment, preventing the etheric body from taking hold of it and failing to take its place properly within the total organism with the help of the higher components. When a tumour forms 'all kinds of external influences gain ready access'; the physical body subjects itself to 'external nature, which is inimical to man'.

The 'external influences' in question are particularly destructive when they have dropped out of their natural context. Science and culture become materialistic, technological developments proceed apace, and human beings find themselves increasingly surrounded by an environment which invades their being like a foreign element. Among these influences are foodstuffs which have been heavily denatured.

At first functional disorders develop in the metabolism, but in the long run these foreign elements cause some cells to extricate themselves from the overall order of the body. They then begin to multiply very fast, thus causing a tumour to form. The total intake of proteins, fats, sugar and minerals in foods should be considered in this light, since they become foreign elements if they cannot be controlled by the organism.

All food is to some extent a foreign element which introduces a certain heaviness into the organism. This heaviness has to be overcome by the etheric body. When there is a tendency to cancer this is often insufficiently achieved and that is why it is so important not to eat more than is necessary. On the whole these days far too much is eaten and the organism has to struggle to come to grips with these excessive amounts.

It is particularly easy to eat too much **protein**, and the organism is then incapable of digesting the proteins sufficiently. They remain as foreign substances and weigh down the physical body. Since they are insufficiently filled with life forces they tend set up a process of putrefaction, especially in the intestines. Rudolf Steiner pointed to this danger long ago in various lectures. More recently Wendt and Schwarz have observed this phenomenon.[4] They relate the toxic effect of too much protein to the development of arterio-sclerosis, but it can also be related to cancer. Zabel has frequently stressed the connection between cancer and the actions of toxins.[5]

What is the upper limit for protein intake? Certainly there can be no general rule. There must be individual variations since every human being has his own protein requirement. Rudolf Steiner once mentioned 20-30 g per day. It seems sensible to assume an upper limit that is somewhat lower than the 70 g per day usually claimed nowadays. Furthermore it is extremely important to take into account the quality of the protein and also its organic relationship to the substances accompanying it, for instance iron.

The fact that cancer patients excrete too little urea, in other words that they retain the products of nitrogen catabolism, is attributed by Zabel[5] to an insufficient mastering of animal protein by the metabolism. Urea arises as a result of digesting meat.

Too much **fat** is as bad as too much protein.

Refined and **denatured foods** also disturb the interplay between the human physical and the etheric body. They lack vitality and are weighed down by sheer physical substance. Yet it is the vitality of the food which activates the etheric forces of the organism. A lively play of etheric forces is necessary if substances are to be grasped and integrated into the total organism, so that a one-sided burdening of the organism, which could lead to a tumour, is avoided altogether.

Burkitt's[6] extensive research points in this direction. He found that wherever native Africans abandoned their natural grain based diet, because they had access to a shop selling the refined foods of industrialized countries, they began to suffer increasingly from diseases of civilization such as cancer.

The vitality of foods is decisively influenced by the **method of their**

cultivation. Heavy doses of mineral fertilizer may indeed lead to increased production of crops which can be made exceedingly attractive with the help of chemical 'improvers', but the coarse material structure of these crops means that the living forces of the cosmos only fill them weakly. The balance between the etheric and physical aspects shifts and the heavy, physical side dominates. This burdens the human organism and promotes the tendency to cancer.

Thus all methods of further processing and preservation should as far as possible be careful of the living etheric forces.

What about **deep freezing**? Are the structures of life modified by it? Preservation by means of low temperatures is based on the concept that cold brings life processes to a standstill, so that certain microscopic organisms and enzymes, which might cause deterioration, are put out of action. However, the sudden shock of extremely cold temperatures leaves its mark on the creative forces of life, transforming them in a particular direction. Pfeiffer's copper chloride crystallization method of investigation reveals shapes which are coarsened and more solid.[7] Comparative experiments have also shown that the structure of the creative forces in deep frozen bread and pastry is dissolved much more rapidly in the digestive processes of the mouth than is the case with products stored at normal temperatures. This demonstrates the loss of nutritional value and shows that low temperatures characteristically cause substances to solidify and become rigid and heavy, thus removing them from their living context.

For this reason it is better to avoid deep-freezing where cancer prevention is the aim.

Irradiation, too, makes foodstuffs more foreign to the human organism. Different countries have different regulations regarding the use of irradiation as a means of preserving foods. Guidelines have been worked out by IAETA and WHO, and now these agencies of the UN are requesting all countries to alter their food legislation correspondingly. Irradiation of foodstuffs is already permitted in some countries as follows:[8]

Canada	potatoes, onions, wheat, flour
Denmark	potatoes
Holland	mushrooms, potatoes, poultry, onions, herbs
Israel	potatoes, onions
Italy	potatoes, onions, garlic
Japan	potatoes
USA	wheat.

In West Germany a problem has arisen in connection with exotic spices. Hitherto they have been sterilized by the use of ethylene oxide, a synthetic gas. This is because for instance pepper or cinnamon can poison vast amounts of foodstuffs if they are infected with pathogens from their countries of origin. Now, however, serious suspicions have arisen that ethylene oxide can cause cancer. Scandinavian countries have already forbidden its use.

So what happens to foodstuffs when they are irradiated? Scientists admit that irradiation acts like a bomb. The genetic material in the cell nucleus is destroyed; bacteria, fungi and insects are killed; aromatic substances and vitamins are partly dissolved and new chemical combinations arise. Some of the latter are toxic, but as the quantities are so minute, many scientists consider them to be negligible. Certainly many generations of experimental animals have eaten food sterilized by irradiation, so far without any damaging side effects. Nevertheless, we must ask: If ethylene oxide, hitherto permitted, can suddenly come to be suspected of producing cancer, might not the same thing happen one day in respect of irradiated foodstuffs? Certainly irradiation denatures foods and makes them more lifeless to a considerable extent. This in itself burdens the human organism in the manner we have come to regard as undesirable in connection with cancer. Let us also not forget that spent rods from nuclear reactors can be used as the source of radiation for the process of irradiating foods!

From all this we can gather that foods grown on healthy soil and processed with the greatest of care are most important in connection with cancer prevention. In such foods the creative etheric forces are strong enough to stimulate the human organism to overcome the heaviness of the physical substances taken in.

Grains (see Chapter 11) coupled with culinary herbs, such as those belonging to the carrot family (Umbelliferae), are especially suited. All further dietary possibilities are discussed in Chapter 12. Here let us mention only one important factor which is usually overlooked: The catabolism of foods in the digestive tract is made considerably easier by the digestive processes which take place in the mouth. Therefore it is important to chew food very thoroughly, to mix it well with saliva and taste it consciously. This is an important aspect of cancer prevention.

3. CANCER-CAUSING FOREIGN SUBSTANCES IN ENVIRONMENT AND FOOD

Increasing notice is being taken of a further factor among the causes of cancer: the rapid growth of cells in reaction to external irritants. It is well-known that a tumour can form in response to constant external irritation, either mechanical or chemical. Bronchial and lung cancer are examples. They arise chiefly as a consequence of the constant irritation caused by the tar derivatives inhaled by the smoker. But a chemical stimulus is not always necessary. In rare cases constant mechanical pressure or friction, such as that caused by a pipe in the corner of the mouth, can suffice.

In recent years a great number of substances which can contribute to cancer have been found in foodstuffs. These are called carcinogens. Little is so far known about how they work. Reliable experimental results are available only with regard to animals. Another problem is that often a number of irritants, a number of carcinogenic substances, work together to cause a tumour.

How do tumours arise as a result of external irritants? Can we find in the knowledge given by Anthroposophy an explanation as to why they should cause a tumour to grow?

An irritation is a process of perception, so it belongs in the sensory area of the organism. An external irritation is perceived, often far below the threshold of consciousness and not always by a familiar sense organ. Yet it is a process of perception taking place within the sphere of the organs. What happens during sense perception? What is typical for a sense organ?

As explained earlier, the physical body is predominant in a sense organ, whereas the other components of man's being are here only loosely connected to the organic realm.

Think of the eye. It provides the soul with a gateway to the world. But it has to contain a device which will ensure that the soul can gain a clear image of its surroundings. Vital forces cannot be permitted to pulse through it nor bring too much blood to it. Instead it is far more like an instrument in physics. Thus the world is reflected in it and a clear image is given. Only at the back of the eye, in the retina, do we find capillary and nerve tissues which collect the sense impressions. Eye and brain together create an image, a picture which is incorporated into the soul. It can be brought to the fore once again in the form of a memory. The link between nerve and blood provides the basis for an immediate reaction to a perception. This reaction belongs to the will and takes place below the threshold of consciousness. The conscious working through of impressions is different; it is one of the tasks most worthy of human beings. We should bear in mind that the more we perceive, the more impressions we have which need to be inwardly assimilated.

People today, particularly in towns, are at the mercy of countless perceptions most of which they cannot even register, let alone work through: advertisements, lights, crowds, street noise, a babel of voices, the mass media, an indecipherable array of odours, and also the huge variety of tastes in food. No wonder we speak of being overwhelmed with impressions. And what are the consequences? Our soul can no longer move about freely at the gateway of the senses; it can no longer breathe freely. All these stimuli impose on us like foreign invaders. And the consequences are not long in coming. Our soul feels oppressed; if it is unable to counter all these external impressions with a powerful, spiritual thought life, it finds itself bound too firmly to material existence.

In the region of the will the reaction at first takes the form of restlessness, aggression, nervousness, sleeplessness. The will shoots out profusely in answer to all this external stimulation. But then another reaction generally takes place. Spirit and soul withdraw. So now the physical forces dominate and the disposition for cancer is born.

Eating involves primarily the sense of taste. But we do not taste only with tongue and palate. Our whole digestive process is based on an unconscious process of tasting. Our intestinal villi 'feel' the chyme; mucous membranes and intestinal glands, and especially liver and pancreas, taste our food. Their reaction, the secretion of juices, depends on what they find. We sense this when we say to what extent a meal agreed with us. In those whose instinct for food is still more or less intact, this usually parallels the way the meal tasted in our mouth.

Once again we must consider the proper ratio of stimulus and reaction. When we eat we take in physical matter which our organism

11

perceives by the sense of taste and with which it has to come to grips. Our organism is adjusted to appreciate foods which have been grown and ripened naturally. But frequently nowadays it is expected to cope with denatured foods and above all with foreign additives. Many of these, as we have seen, are carcinogenic.

How, then, are we to understand the appearance of a carcinoma in this connection? Something Rudolf Steiner said can point the way. He described a tumour as a misplaced sense organ. What he meant was that something which is normal in the sphere of the senses—the predominance of physical matter, as in the eye, which he called a natural camera—provides the basis for a cancerous growth if it takes place in the realm of metabolism, where our etheric body and the higher components of our being ought to permeate intimately the organic and physical structure of our body. (See Chapter 1)

The misplaced creation of a sense organ is provoked when our ego and astral body are overwhelmed by foreign stimuli to an extent that interferes with their ability to perceive. Together with the worn-out etheric forces they withdraw from our body. Then the cells of our body become abnormal because now they are no longer contained within the overall plan of our supersensible components.

An abundance of results of animal experiments are available showing the effects of certain substances in food on the stimulation of cancerous growths. In a number of cases researchers succeeded in producing the tumour as a result of a mix of several carcinogenic substances. Here are a few examples, with apologies for the unavoidable chemical terms.

First we have *Aspergillus* mildew with its content of aflatoxins. Peanuts are frequently affected. The highly toxic substances invade not only the fruits but also products made from them. Animals fed with these suffered severe liver disease and pigs contracted cancer of the liver. Epidemiological research indicates that humans, too, are sensitive to aflatoxins.

Nitrosamines can also be counted among the carcinogenic substances. They arise when nitrite reacts with secondary amines. Resulting from the use of nitrate as a fertilizer, such substances are now present in nature and can even appear in drinking water. Norwegian fish meal, for which nitrite is used as a preservative, was found to contain a good deal of nitrosamine. Nitrosamines also arise in warmed-up spinach containing nitrate as a result of having been cultivated with nitrogenous fertilizer. The smoking of foodstuffs can also lead to the formation of carcinogenic aromatic hydrocarbons. Benzopyrenes, for instance, have been found in mutton and fish. Grilling sausages, can lead to the formation of carcinogenic substances. Considerable amounts were found in sausages barbecued over pine cones. None of these foods by itself could be termed a cause for cancer, but people on normal diets today are exposed to not inconsiderable amounts of carcinogenic substances.

It is difficult to say which of the countless additives used in foods today might be carcinogenic. This is not least because the available data stem almost exclusively from animal experiments which have limited applicability to human beings. Also in today's overall toxicological situation many separate substances come together, some forming new compounds. These might be more toxic than the original compounds which have been tested.

For these reasons it is best to avoid all additives so widely used for preservation, prevention of mildew or simply to improve appearance, and so on. This includes synthetic substances said to be identical with those occurring naturally. The chemical structure of these substances is indeed identical with that of the products which occur in nature. Thus carotene with an identical formula to that found in carrots can be synthetically produced. These substances are declared to be identical with natural products and may therefore be added without question or any special indication to yogurt, pastries, creme fillings and so on. Consumers ought to arm themselves with as much information as possible.

4. DISORDERS OF THE FLUID ORGANISM ABNORMAL ETHERIC GROWTH FORCES GENERATE CELL PROLIFERATION

Tomatoes, Potatoes, Fungi (Mushrooms), Meat

It is possible for certain types of tissue to be alienated from the organism through being taken over by the realm in which the heaviness of physical forces dominates. But it is also the case that every cell has a tendency to 'do its own thing', which means that it must constantly be called to order and incorporated into the totality of the organism by the superior formative forces. Where there is a predisposition for cancer, cells threaten to slip from the grasp of these forces and lead their own disorganized life.

The vehicle through which the etheric creative forces work is the fluid organism. This is the source of all the physical structures such as the cells of the supportive and connective tissues and of the organs. Thus the solid physical part of the organism is closely allied to the fluid part which serves the etheric forces.

In the earlier chapters we saw the heaviness of the physical body which has subjected itself to influences from its environment as the cause of a cancerous growth. Now let us turn to the fluid organism and the creative forces which work through it. Later we shall also consider the organisms of air, light and warmth in the way they give expression to ego and astral body. So far as cancer is concerned, decisive impulses, either pathological or healing, can emanate from all these realms.

The fluid organism is in constant pulsating motion. Water streams rhythmically not only in the system of heart and circulation but also in all tissues, for instance muscles or brain. Stillness and stagnation never occur. Even the fluid tied up in the cells is in constant exchange with its surroundings. Gerhard Schmidt[9] quotes a modern scientist who speaks of the 'inconceivable intensity' of this exchange: 'Every second billions of water molecules and substances in solution pass in one direction or another through the walls of the capillaries and

14

the membranes which enclose every one of our cells.'

Because of this exchange, the concentration of minerals in our tissue fluids remains constant all the time. For instance the potassium level is always 200 mg per litre of body fluid. Even the minutest fluctuations can lead to life-threatening conditions such as heart failure. Since the potassium content of our food varies considerably, an extremely sensitive interchange is essential.

The same goes for other elements such as sodium, calcium, magnesium, iron, sulphur, phosphorus. They too are dissolved and transformed in the rhythmically moving fluid which is the medium through which they can perform their functions in our organism.

The ratio of potassium to sodium in the body is constant and it is extremely important for a person's health that this ratio should remain undisturbed. In nutrition we ought to bear this in mind. The amount of potassium in our food always demands a corresponding amount of common salt, and vice versa. But in our eating habits today we tend to disregard it. Usually too much salt is taken, up to 10-15 g per day, instead of 5-7.5g. Salt consumption is bumped up above all by the use of tinned and processed foods such as smoked meats and the like. On the other hand when the water in which vegetables or fruit have been cooked is thrown away, there are losses of potassium, and this enhances the effect of high salt consumption.

In cancer, the function of the cells is disturbed in a number of ways. Thus one of the important factors in this illness is the mineral balance and also the dynamism of the fluid organism which serves the exchange of substances. Cell respiration, which we shall be discussing in more detail in a later chapter, is particularly dependent on the catalysts and respiratory enzymes such as iron and magnesium which are bound up in the watery element.

To enliven the fluid organism and stimulate the exchange of substances between blood, tissue fluids and organ cells we can recommend the drinking of liquids in which grains have been boiled, vegetable broths and fruit juices, because of their mineral content. Of all the grains, rice has the most favourable effect on the water balance. An occasional day on which only rice is eaten has proved useful for stimulating the elimination of excess fluid.

Having considered the fluid organism, let us return to the etheric creative forces in the human being, which, as we have seen, are closely linked with the circulation of fluid. These forces give the impulse for cell metabolism and also for cell growth. This cell growth has to conform to the nature of the total organism. But in cancer certain groups of cells grow wildly, without concern for the wellbeing of the totality, exerting tremendous power.

Foods can assist these pathological tendencies in the human organism. It is therefore necessary to ask whether there exist in the plant world any one-sided tendencies in the way things grow which might, if eaten repeatedly, stimulate the uncontrolled growth of cells.

Tomatoes

Rudolf Steiner banned tomatoes for cancer patients and also from any diet aimed at cancer prevention. In order to understand this, let us look at the nature of this fruit.

Like the potato, the tomato is a plant of the deadly nightshade family. This is a family of doubtful reputation, for very many of its members are poisonous, some exceedingly. Many come from the Americas, for example the very toxic thorn-apple, as well as tobacco, sweet peppers, tomatoes and potatoes. In Europe, two poisonous plants have always been particularly feared: deadly nightshade itself, and also henbane. Yet the physician's art can turn them into healing substances, for these two are important medicinal plants.

The name 'nightshade', coupled with their Latin designation 'Solanaceae' (sol = sun), points to an interplay between light and darkness and hints at an abnormality in this interplay.

In earlier times the Latin name of the tomato was *Solanum lycopersicum*. In the sixteenth century it was brought from the warm climes of Peru and Mexico to Europe where it was suspected of being poisonous, and thus disregarded as a food. When it first arrived it was called 'apple of gold' or 'love-apple'. Not until the twentieth century did it suddenly become a generally accepted food. The Latin name was then changed to *Lycopersicum esculentum, 'esculentum'* meaning 'edible'. It seems that this fact had to be particularly emphasized.

Most noticeable about the tomato plant—and typical of all the deadly nightshade family—is the way light and warmth cause its lush, luxuriant growth which does not cease when the flowers begin to form. Even the fruiting parts can produce new shoots. Special measures have to be taken to stem this uncontrolled new growth. The shining red fruits come in many shapes; there are apple, pear or egg-shaped tomatoes, and also the tiny cherry tomatoes. Fruit formation is lush, but the plant lacks the ability to support itself. It is either allowed to grow along the ground or propped up with stakes. It has unpaired

16

pinnate leaves which exude a dull, musty smell.

The property of rank growth would in itself be insufficient indication of a tendency to promote the development of a cancerous tumour. But the tomato also possesses another property which was pointed out by Rudolf Steiner in his 'Agricultural Course'.[10] The tomato plant tends to separate itself off from any living connection with its environment; it is independent of anything else and does not leave the sphere of its own creative forces. Expression is given to this by the fact that the best compost for tomato plants is one which is made of tomato plants. They dislike a well-prepared and matured compost because they feel invaded by creative forces which do not belong to them. Instead they grow well on any kind of rubbish, or animal manure such as guano, which has not been prepared in any way and is therefore still entirely within the realm of physical substance.

Rudolf Steiner applies this image of the tomato to the human being. 'Eating tomatoes', he says, 'has a strong effect on anything in the organism which inclines to encapsulate itself and take on an existence of its own. Therefore—I would like to say this in parenthesis—anyone suffering from a carcinoma should be forbidden to eat tomatoes. For by their very nature tomatoes strongly affect something which works independently in the organism, separating itself off and becoming specialized.'

Recent research has revealed that in unripe tomatoes the alkaloid content (tomatine and solanin) is comparatively high, and that a constant intake of these amounts can lead to arthritis, rheumatism and cancer. This confirms, from another angle, Rudolf Steiner's statement. Consider what quantities of not quite ripe tomatoes are eaten all the year round nowadays!

Potatoes

Directly after describing these characteristics of tomatoes, Rudolf Steiner mentions potatoes: 'Potatoes resemble tomatoes to some extent in this connection. They, too, work in a strongly independent way.'

However, he does not relate this separation from the totality of the organism, as he does in the case of the tomato, to the organic process of tumour formation. When eaten, he says, the potato causes the functioning of certain parts of the brain to be separated from the totality of the organism and made independent. Materialistic thinking is the consequence of this. Its increase began in the nineteenth century when

17

the excessive consumption of potatoes started. We cannot go into this in more detail here, except to say that the similar effect of the potato is indeed related to the purpose of this book but belongs in the field of embryology.

Rudolf Steiner says that the consumption of potatoes by the expectant mother causes the physical embryo to grow dense in a way which makes it difficult for the soul of the child and its spiritual individuality, coming gradually down towards incarnation, to penetrate the body. Thus once again we see the phenomenon of a physical organism making itself independent, excluding a superior spiritual element and succumbing to the earthly forces of solidification and heaviness.

Potatoes and grains are compared by Rudolf Steiner in this connection. He points out that the ears of corn take in the forces of the sun's light and warmth as they ripen. 'The plant is approached by the spirit here. The spirit shows affinity. So when the spirit and soul of the child encounter in the womb something that has been built up with the help of nourishment made from grains, they can work easily. But if they encounter an embryonic head which has been formed chiefly with the help of food containing potatoes, then the spirit cannot work in a healing way.'

Embryonic malformations arising as a result of the mother's consumption of potatoes are reminiscent of the appearance presented by a carcinoma.

Of course we shall not go so far as to count potatoes among the foods which cause cancer, but we do exclude them from the diet of cancer patients and recommend, when cancer prevention is the aim, that they are only eaten sparingly. In the same way Rudolf Steiner warns: 'Potato consumption should not be overdone.' The abnormality of the processes that give rise to potatoes is also evident from the fact that they form their typical toxin (solanin) when exposed to the forces of light.[11]

Fungi (Mushrooms) and Algae

In addition to potatoes and tomatoes, fungi and algae are not recommended for cancer patients. They grow hastily, have no relationship light, and have a tendency to toxic decomposition.[12] In this they resemble malignant tumours. Furthermore, they belong to the far past of the earth's evolution and are thus not compatible with man's nutritional needs today. They are not part of present-day evolution. The gelling agent agar agar is one of the algae in question.

Meat

Meat brings many problems with it. First there is the very questionable quality of the meat available. Intensive rearing of stock is opposed to the true nature of the animals. Every measure undertaken is founded on the necessity for financial competition. Apart from food concentrates, the animals are treated with medicines and hormones which promote meat production. One drastic example recently aired in the European press is the content of oestrogens, female hormones, in veal. Meat containing such growth hormones has its effect on human beings and the very thing it is likely to spark off is the uncontrolled growth of cells in the human organism. (See Chapter 12)

The etheric creative forces can be snatched from their proper order in another way too. Rudolf Steiner describes[13] the way in which growth and formative forces work in early childhood to form the body's organs but are later, through the right kind of education, transformed into the forces of thought and memory. In the normal run of this process the organs gain a healthy form and structure. But if the transformation fails to take place properly, some of the forces which should have formed the organs are held back; they remain as islands of congested growth forces which do not conform to the order of the total organism but can instead degenerate into the formation of new structures. 'If the normal amount of organizing forces is transformed at the change of teeth, then the amount left in the organism for later life is exactly that required to shape and maintain its structure in a normal way. But if too few are transformed, then superfluous forces remain below and can later make their appearance anywhere, forming new growths which are carcinomas.'

These congested growth forces, having failed to become transformed into memory forces during childhood, and which under certain circumstances can lead to the formation of malignant new growths, require a diet which does not encourage excessive growth. From this point of view, too, the intake of protein should be reduced. Also, instead of fresh milk, soured and fermented milk products are to be preferred. Fresh milk may be compared with a hormone, and sour milk with a vitamin.

19

5. THE CANCER CELL FAILS TO BREATHE

Respiratory Function and Nutrition

Every normal cell breathes; air streams through it. The cell takes in the oxygen with the help of which it performs its metabolic process. In physiology the comparison to a process of combustion is often used.

The circulation of fluid—we spoke of a fluid organism—is impregnated by a superior system of forces, the etheric body. Similarly the supply of air—from that of the lungs right into the cell tissues—is determined by a totality of forces. We can speak in this connection of an airy organism which has form, is in motion and has infrastructure. And whereas water embodies the life-forming principle, air allows an element of soul to enter into the organic world. Living organisms which breathe in oxygen are beings with a soul. Even the ancient Greeks had the idea that with the inhaled air the human being was taking into himself something that had the quality of a soul. They called it 'pneuma'.

This 'something with the quality of a soul'—Rudolf Steiner called it the astral body (see Chapter 1)—breathes throughout every part of the organism. It integrates every single cell into the totality of the organism. And the soul of the human being can express itself in every organ and in every function of the body, using them as the basis for its activity on earth. Cancer cells cut themselves off from this. They do not breathe or take in oxygen; in a way they suffocate.

This menacing lack could have come about in one of two ways. Either too little air was supplied to the cells in the first place. Or they were incapable of taking in oxygen, perhaps because of a lack of respiratory enzymes. Often these two factors cannot be easily distinguished.

Let us start with the first factor, inadequate breathing. The process of breathing affects every single cell. And wherever the air organism is at work, the astral body is active. An interesting study has underlined the importance of deep breathing in the field of cancer prevention. One hundred and twenty members of an association of older long-distance runners agreed to run 5 km daily. Over a period of five years there was not one case of cancer amongst them, although they were all at the critical age for developing cancer.

Inadequate breathing is a widespread evil of our time. There are many causes. Lack of exercise in the open air leads to the habit of shallow breathing. Air pollution in cities also leads to shallow breathing. Some people hold in their breath in a cramped way because of the stress of modern life, or they do not dare to breathe out because their soul is oppressed by some unconscious anxiety. Others breathe out too much because exhaustion causes everything to flow out of them.

All these forms of breathing inadequacy bring disorder into the whole of the air organism. And this in turn disturbs cell respiration. Breathing is released and stimulated by soul hygiene, by artistic activities, especially in music, speech and eurythmy. All these measures are beneficial to cell respiration and thus constitute an important element in cancer prevention.

D. Warburg was awarded the Nobel Prize for his research into cell respiration. He discovered all the biochemical processes involved. With the help of respiratory enzymes, the oxygen brought by the blood is used for the combustion of sugars, which are also constantly being supplied to the cells. In this way the energy for cell metabolism is obtained. It is important that the sugar reserves in the cells are totally burnt up. Scientists call this aerobic respiration. It is the way every normal cell in the body breathes.

But this is not so in the case of cancer cells. They do not absorb oxygen, in other words they do not breathe. They gain their energy through breaking down sugars by fermentation leading to the formation of lactic acid. This anaerobic respiration, which is actually not respiration at all, is done outside the human organism by primitive cells such as yeast cells. Warburg used these for his studies. Cancer cells produce substances which destroy the respiratory enzymes of normal cells. These can then no longer breathe and must either perish or turn to fermentation instead. Cancer cells, which gain their energy without using oxygen, are capable of doing this already and continue to spread.

The abnormal cell metabolism in the cancer patient is not confined to the cancer cells alone but involves the whole organism. Warburg observed an increased readiness to ferment in the red blood corpuscles of cancer patients. This shows how important nutrition is, for it influences the total human being.

The aim of nutrition as a therapy and as a preventative measure must therefore be to activate cell respiration, to stimulate the supply of oxygen to the cells, and to discourage fermentative metabolism. It must not be forgotten that pesticides, tar products, and also other carcinogenic substances, can block the functions of the respiratory catalysts.

How can the production of respiratory enzymes be stimulated by means of nutrition? One special group of foods are those containing red pigments. Their pigmentation comes from anthocyanes which have active oxygen groups. The patient can take them in the juices of bilberries (blueberries), black currants, cherries and red grapes. A clinic in Hungary used beetroot to achieve remarkable success with a considerable number of cancer and leukaemia patients. The cure has to be applied intensively for a considerable time. The juice of 1 kg of freshly squeezed beetroots must be taken daily, spread over the day; or alternatively, if available, half a litre of lactic-fermented[15] beetroot juice. In addition large amounts of root vegetables should be eaten, and it is advantageous if they are available in lactic-fermented form too. A chemical finding points in the same direction: Lactic-fermented foods stimulate the production of vitamin B_2 in the intestine. This is a component of the riboflavin in the cells. It is needed for oxygen exchange.

W. Zabel[5] has pointed out that cell respiration can be stimulated by the intake of fats containing a high proportion of the unsaturated fatty acids linoleic acid and linolenic acid. This is understandable, since these fatty acids exhibit free bonds which they seek to saturate with oxygen, thus stimulating internal respiration. However, they should be used only in the form of cold—pressed oils and may not be heated. To mix them with quark is a useful method, since this makes it easier for the organism to absorb them.

Plants breathe most intensively in their leaves, where substances are formed which stimulate similar processes in the human organism. Green-leaved salads are therefore a must. If possible buy biodynamically or organically grown lettuce and other salad vegetables, for the use of cultivation methods such as silica sprays stimulates the dynamic processes in the leaves. This may be observed even in the more luminous green of the leaves.

Cell respiration also depends on certain trace elements, especially iron and magnesium. Regular consumption of sufficient whole-grain

22

foods and bread ensure the proper intake for the human organism.

Lactic-fermented vegetables have an important place in nutrition for cancer patients. Kuhl[14] introduced them as a cancer diet and since then they have been used with much success.

They work on the metabolism and their effect seems to be non-specific, lying simply in the stimulation and regulation of the digestive process. In the stomach, where in cancer patients gastric secretions are often abnormal, lactic-fermented foods help to increase the production of hydrochloric acid and also to decrease any acid excesses. Stimulation of the pancreas relieves the strain on all the other digestive organs. Lactose fermenting bacteria bind putrefaction not only in the food but also in the intestine. A healthy intestinal milieu is created and the intestinal flora are improved. This can be very helpful, since all cancers come about on the basis of metabolic disorders.

Over and above this, lactic-fermented foods can be assumed to to have a beneficial effect on the actual tumour. How can this be?

As we have said, in normal cell metabolism oxygen is used for the combustion of sugars. A supersensible process is connected with this aspect of the breathing process, for the astral body plays its part wherever oxygen is breathed in, guiding the process and preventing the sugar from fermenting. Instead it is entirely converted in the breathing, giving rise to energy which is used by the organism. If fermentation takes place, lactic acid is produced. This can be found in the body wherever sugar metabolism takes place anaerobically, that is without oxygen. Physiologically it is created in muscles as glycogen is split while the muscle is working. Muscle pain and stiffness after exercise is the result of an accumulation of lactic acid.

Normal cell respiration also always produces traces of lactic acid, but this is straight away taken back into the metabolic process through the respiratory process. The higher components of man's being are called upon to intervene in order to immediately reverse the production of lactic acid.[15]

This indicates that lactic acid stimulates the processes of cell respiration. So we can understand why Rudolf Steiner recommended the lactic acid injections for cancer patients. It challenges the organism to come to grips with the processes of cell respiration.

The importance of lactic-fermented products in the diet of cancer patients is to be seen in the same light (see Chapter 12). If the cancer patient eats lactic-fermented vegetables, the lactic acid they contain does not increase the fermentation processes. On the contrary, the normal lactic acid process, which leads directly to respiratory conversion, is stimulated, thus making possible the transition to normal cell respiration.

A diet which makes use of sprouted seeds has a similar effect. During the process of germination the seed contains a maximum of lactic acid. In a damp, dark environment, without light or air, the plant uses up the nutritional substances of the seed. The process is one of fermentation. Think of the first line in Rudolf Steiner's table grace: 'The plant seeds are quickened in the night of the earth.' Then in the second line we hear: 'The green herbs are sprouting through the might of the air.' Now air is taken in, oxygen is added, and fermentation is replaced by breathing. The potential produced by the germinating plant can be used as a dietary measure to improve abnormal cell respiration.

Something different is sparked off by the habitual consumption of products containing sugar and white flour. Cells whose respiration is weak cannot cope with a high intake of sugar and are thus forced into fermentation leading to carcinomatous changes. These products, which anyway do not belong in a wholefood diet, should be totally avoided by those with a predisposition to cancer. In the case of whole-grain products, on the other hand, the carbohydrate is metabolized slowly, so high blood sugar levels, and the accompanying dangerous flooding of the cells with sugar, do not arise.

6. DISORDERS OF LIGHT METABOLISM IN CANCER PATIENTS

The Light Quality of Foods

Light is closely linked to the element of air. The air is illumined by light. Just as air in the human being is organized and differentiated to form an 'air organism' in which the astral body works, so is it also with light. Principles of structure and form are present in light and these work into the movement of air in the organism. Rudolf Steiner says:[16] 'Light shares in organizing every part of the air organism. With air, light lives in the human being.'

In the previous chapter the inability of cancer cells to breathe was described. Now we come to the fact that they also exclude themselves from the metabolism of light. The cancer cell lies in the darkness. This is interesting in the context of comprehensive cancer prevention, both dietary and therapeutic.

Light streams into the human being through sense organs and skin, but also through the food eaten. Apart from the visible, optical aspect, light also has an energy component. It has been found that light has a stimulating effect on all kinds of living processes such as the water balance, protein, fat and sugar metabolism, blood formation, the circulation, thyroid and adreno-cortical function as well as the sexual cycle and its secondary characteristics. In addition everyone knows how light affects people's soul life.

Light metabolism is regulated by a higher principle, the astral body, also called the light body. This belongs to the realm of soul and spirit but lives in constant interplay with the organic functions already described.

The inner nature of this light body can be experienced if external sight is extinguished. A blind man, Jacques Lusseyran, possessed this capacity to a unique extent. He could use his light body as an organ of perception for living creatures in his environment. He could sense plant life and had clear perceptions, for instance, of trees as he passed them, and even of the surrounding landscape over long distances. He also perceived what emanated from the characters and souls of human beings. But the capacity was extinguished when his own soul was darkened by bad temper, antipathy or impatience.[17]

So the inner light body is touched on two sides; on the one hand by the light of the soul, and on the other by the light that streams into the organism through the senses and through food. Contact with the external world stimulates an internal activity which leads to the creation of an 'inner' light which belongs to the human individuality. The same takes place in all nutritional processes. External substances are not taken in and transformed into the body's own substance. Instead, food activates the organism to work in such a way that new substance is created. Similarly the external, 'foreign' light is at first broken down and extinguished. Then inner activity starts which leads to all the many organic functions we have described. To take this into account, the scientific concept of the 'energy component' of light will have to be extended. Herbert Sieweke says on this: 'Just as the human being maintains a process by which substance comes into being, stimulating and kindling it by taking in food, so does he also bring about a light-forming process which is triggered by actively receiving the external world of light.'[18]

The various activities set in motion by the intake of light are part of the regulatory system of the human light organism, which works right into the organic functions and structures.

What conclusions can we draw with regard to cancer prevention? Since the disorder usually develops over many years, preventative measures are desirable, measures which will stimulate the metabolism of light.

There are three ways to do this: firstly by taking in light through the sense organs, avoiding long periods in artificial light, especially neon light; secondly by opening one's soul to all that is light and beautiful; and finally by eating food which has a high light quality. The present book is concerned with the third point.

How does light work in the plants we use as food? It is worrying to see how the cultivated landscapes of Europe are gradually losing their light forces. The landscapes flooded with light we used to know have disappeared. Many meadow flowers have gone and many species of butterfly are missing. All sorts of birds, too, have withdrawn from our latitudes. This situation makes the cultivation of the land with mineral fertilizers, monocultures, and also the use of poisons, all the more grave. The only hope for improvement lies in a proper care

26

of the environment by working the soil with organic methods.

The bio-dynamic method employs a silica preparation which is sprayed on the green leaves of the plants during their vegetative period. This improves the light quality of the produce, for silica helps living creatures to open up to the light. In human skin and sense organs, too, in keeping with their function, we find subtle amounts of silica. The effectiveness of this silica preparation has been proved in a number of comparative studies and shows itself especially in the formation of high-quality protein.

Rudolf Steiner has given us some interesting details about the nature of the light body. He describes quite concretely how impulses of soul and spirit cause 'seeds of light' to shine out in the human organism: 'Moral ideals which stimulate the warmth organism cause sources of light to come into being in the air organism. By being capable of enthusiasm for moral ideals, the human being bears a source of light within himself.' Such an insight can become a bridge to enable us to understand the connection between the spiritual and the physical aspects of the human being, for the sources of light springing up in the soul realm have a bearing on numerous physical processes.

On the other hand, almost all organic processes generate light effects. This is being investigated by a new branch of science, biophoton research. With the help of measuring instruments it has been found that normal cell-division is always accompanied by a most delicate light radiation. This is described as a mitochondrial radiation because it has to do with the mitochondria, which are important cell-elements connected with cell-division. But organic complexes such as the nervous system also send out light rays even though no cell-division or reproduction is involved. Circulating blood does the same, and the intensity varies with different illnesses. Thus the blood of a tuberculosis patient sends out mighty rays. As we know, in tuberculosis the metabolism of light is disturbed. Cancer cells, on the other hand, withdraw from any work with light. They grow in the dark. When they divide, no rays of light are emitted. Research into this has been conducted in an institute in Moscow.[19] A German radiologist, A. Popp, has also described the radiation of the cancer cell as something that looks as if it has been extinguished in comparison with that of a healthy cell. He suggests that this phenomenon could be a useful tool for the early diagnosis of cancer.[20]

The amount of light sent out by plants can be directly measured. There is a clear difference between produce grown by organic and by conventional methods. In an article published in the the magazine *Zeitschrift für Naturheilverfahren* (Magazine for Natural Medicine) we read: 'On the basis of the ultra-weak photon emission of biological systems a method has been developed which permits the objective measurement of the biological condition of plants. Significant differences in the photon emission of plants were found to depend on the conditions of their cultivation (e.g. fertilizers used).'

Cells extracted from the juices of vegetables (carrots, celeriac, beetroot) grown by different methods were investigated by this procedure. Without exception in blind trials the plants grown by organic methods were found to differ significantly from those cultivated by 'modern' or conventional methods. In seed grain, too, there was an equally clear difference in quality.[20]

The forces of the light ether bound by food plants are released in the human organism during digestion. In the above—mentioned Gurvich Institute in Moscow it has been found that a particularly large amount of light rays emanate from the contents of the small intestine. Rudolf Steiner made a statement which corroborates this.[19]

As has already been said, this freed etheric light has to be transformed within the human organism, for to start with it corresponds to the nature of the original plant. This brings about processes in the organism which generate light the intensity of which depends on the quality of the food plant eaten. Here we arrive at the significance of the right diet for cancer patients, whose cell tissues urgently need increased activity of the light organism.

So special emphasis must be placed on produce grown by the biodynamic method. And preference should be given to silica plants such as grains, and also green-leaf vegetables and salads, and fruits such as apples. Culinary herbs rich in essential oils and resins are also valuable light-bearers. Carrots show their relationship to light by their orange colour. And finally good-quality cooking and salad oils may be mentioned as light bearing foods.

7. THE CANCER CELL AS A COLD FOCUS

Stimulating the Warmth Organism by Nutrition

Like light, air and fluids, warmth is in constant inner motion in the human organism. This warmth organism, too, is formed, differentiated and given limits by a higher spiritual principle. We saw in the previous chapters that the etheric body organizes the fluid element, and the astral body the air and light elements. In the same way the warmth element is organized by the human ego, which collects, shapes and structures it into a warmth organism. The ego finds an entry to man's bodily aspect through the medium of warmth. Without taking into account the way the ego enters in through warmth it is not possible to understand how spirit, soul and body can work in harmony together.

The activity of the warmth element is kindled by enthusiasm for moral goals such as the ideals of benevolence, freedom, kindness, truth. Theoretical ideas, on the other hand, chill the warmth organism. Always it is a question of how the ego can find its way to the will. Warmth, the movement of the blood, and will impulses are all of a kind and belong together.

Physical exercise also stimulates the creation of warmth, and so does the consumption of food, as we shall describe.

In the cancer patient the capacity of the warmth organism to react is weakened. Therefore the ego lacks the possibility of actively entering fully into the organism. So the cancer cells succeed in separating themselves off. They lack warmth and form a cold focus. They escape from the rulership of the ego which manifests via warmth and gives direction to all the body's processes and structures both as a whole and individually. Then the cancer cells proliferate under their own steam, taking no account of the totality. They bring about anarchy which leads to the destruction of the state.

Because of the feebleness of their warmth organism, people who are disposed towards cancer hardly ever react with a temperature to colds or infections. One aspect of cancer prevention is therefore to ensure that even in childhood and youth the capacity of the warmth organism to be active is stimulated. Acute feverish attacks must not be stifled but allowed to run their course. Only natural treatments such as water applications (cool compresses) should be used. Antibiotics should be avoided. Clothes made from natural materials also help the body's warmth to be regulated properly.

Once a tumour has manifested, temperature reactions in the organism can be stimulated by hyperthermal baths (Lampert). Injections of mistletoe also bring about a rise in temperature. As Rudolf Steiner put it, a mantle of warmth forms around the tumour, in some cases bringing about regression or even putting an end to further growth.

Nutrition can also be used to stimulate the warmth organism. This is very important both in cancer prevention and also as a basis for therapy in the case of a manifest tumour. So we have to take account of the warmth quality of foods.

Warmth is an attribute of something living. There is no life without warmth. In the eternal snow and ice of the earth's polar regions no life can develop. In the realm of all that lives, warmth manifests as an aspect of the etheric creative forces. This is also called the 'warmth ether'. Earthly fire destroys, brings about disintegration. In contrast, the warmth ether leads life into the manifest world, causes organic forms to arise and mature in a rhythmically ordered way, each in its own time. It works together with the other ethers, those of the solid, fluid and airy elements.

If the warmth ether is to stimulate and ripen plants, in the right way, their various components must be in harmony with one another. When chemical fertilizers are used, growth is too lush so that the substance of the plant becomes too compact and cannot ripen properly. This impairs the warmth quality of the produce, for in the process of ripening the warmth ether enters the substance of the plant and remains bound there. The bio-dynamic method of soil and plant cultivation ensures that the plant becomes sensitive to cosmic influences and opens up to the warmth ether which streams in. The produce then has a high 'warmth quality'.

When it is digested by the human being its warmth ether is freed and stimulates the warmth processes in the body. This clarifies for us the relationship between cancer and the quality of foods. It is easy to understand that foods with a dynamic warmth quality stimulate corresponding processes in the human organism, thus counteracting the tendency to form tumours, whereas produce grown with mineral fertilizers only burdens the warmth organism.

It is not a question of food being nice and hot, though this too can be of value. We are speaking here of an inner warmth quality which is frequently destroyed by cooking. In this sense raw vegetables and salads can have a higher warmth quality than cooked food, since they stimulate the body to produce more warmth of its own.

On the other hand, ice-cold drinks and foods can irritate the warmth organism. But what about **deep frozen** produce? Should we not assume that the warmth ether is affected by an invasion of extremely low temperatures and that food thus treated could lead to disorders of the subtle processes in the human organism? Those who are in good health can counteract this, of course. But what if the body is repeatedly expected to cope?[21]

Grains are closely related to the warmth organism in the human body. So they are the most suitable food for human beings. Millet especially stimulates the production of warmth. The medieval abbot Ekkehard of St Gall gave the blessing: 'May millet not give you fever and heat!' In those days feverish illnesses were feared as the scourge of mankind. Nowadays, in contrast, people suffer from being unable to generate a raised temperature. This is especially so in those with a tendency to cancer. For them the opposite blessing would be good: 'May millet give you warmth and fever!' In this sense, grains are foods which work against cancer, whole grain flours of course, not white flour.

Fats have the task of generating warmth in the human organism. Those suitable must be high in unsaturated fatty acids which are volatile and metabolize easily. They do not deposit themselves in the cells of the body but are permanently evaporating in a kind of combustion process, thus bringing about the creation of warmth. Droplets of fat have been found in cancer cells. This is a sign that the process has been blocked so that the generation of warmth is upset.

Among the **herbs** indigenous to Europe, the Labiatae are particularly disposed to warm the metabolism. So we should take care to flavour our food with them. Basil, marjoram, rosemary, hyssop, thyme—to name only a few—are very versatile in their use. The Umbelliferae, too, are bearers of warmth. An expression of this is that their seeds contain oil—for example caraway and dill. We may also add spices from warm countries, for instance turmeric, ginger and nutmeg.

31

The warmth quality of plants comes to fullest maturity in fruits and seeds. In sun-ripened apples, pears, peaches or soft fruits delightful aromatic substances are formed which are an expression of the working of warmth. Ripeness is a precondition for good warmth quality. Unfortunately, for reasons of transport and storage, fruits are nearly always harvested nowadays before they are fully ripe.

Additives and chemicals set up a dangerous barrier against the living flow of warmth forces. Often they cause the formation of cold foci and thus promote a disposition to cancer.

Once again, an effective prophylaxis with regard to cancer is the maintenance of the human being's warmth organism and its functioning by means of carefully selected foods.

8. SILICA PROCESSES WHICH PROVIDE FORM

Filling the Form with Light and Warmth

To counteract cancer cells, which proliferate without shape or form and fail to adapt to the pattern of the human being, it is necessary both to activate formative forces and to ease their task of moulding the human organism. In order to do their work, formative forces need earthly substances which help them to stimulate certain processes. Silica is a substance which serves the process of moulding shape and form. In its pure state we know it as translucent, six-sided rock crystal. Organically it appears bound to oxygen as silicic acid by means of which it supports the plant and works in the delicate structures. Cereals with their structured ears and beards are typical silica plants, 70-80% of whose ash consists of silicic acid. In the animal kingdom, too, the most delicate filigree shapes, such as those of the radiolaria in the ocean, are created with the help of this substance.

Light also needs a substance through which it can work in the organic realm and it, too, makes use above all of silica, though also of magnesium and iron.

The human organism is interlaced with a delicate framework of silicic acid. This is concentrated more in the skin, enveloping us in a kind of silica cloak. On the one hand it acts as a protection; but on the other it prevents us from becoming 'thick-skinned', helping us to use our skin as an organ with which to make contact with the outside world. In the same way our sense organs are shaped by silica, especially our eyes, though as described elsewhere, hardly any life forces flow through the eyes, for they function almost like a physical apparatus. The human ego must be allowed to pass unhindered and uninfluenced through the eyes in order to unite itself with whatever object it wants to perceive.

In the metabolic realm the situation is different. Here life pulses through all the organs as blood and fluids flow through them. Substances such as silica are constantly dissolving and reforming. This

33

dynamic process makes it possible for formative forces to intervene in the material world, organizing tissues in accordance with their own pattern. Every part of the organism is individually formed, and all human beings have their own individual bodily shape, whether it be their nose or the palms of their hands, or their brain, liver or kidneys. It is the silica process which makes this possible.

The fetal membranes enveloping the human embryo are especially rich in silicic acid. The form to be created here is not only that of the human being in general but also that of a particular individual.

The process of tumour formation comes about when the human form is unable to manifest fully in the body. To re-open the way for a full manifestation, we must endeavour to activate silica processes.

As rock crystals show so impressively, silica is translucent. In a way it is a door through which light, and with it warmth, can stream in. This applies not only to the intercourse of the human organism with its environment. Within the organism, too, light and warmth circulate constantly in an orderly way, and they need silica in order to be able to unite with the material world. Silica is not present in a crude, substantial form, but finely potentized, like a homoeopathically diluted medicine.

Silica is also used in this way in bio-dynamic agriculture. Whereever the light and warmth organisms are to function properly they need healthy silica dynamics.[22]

What foods stimulate the silica processes in the human organism? First of all we may note that produce grown by the bio-dynamic method contains more silica than that grown by conventional methods. In cereals even when the ears are fully ripe, and therefore no longer connected to the soil by the stream of substances, the silica content continues to increase.

So cereals may be called silica plants. Their finely-chiselled shapes and their relationship with light and warmth bear witness to this, as does chemical analysis, which shows that they contain 70-80% silica. Millet, rye and barley contain most of all. Millet is therefore a useful addition to the diet in cases of skin disorders in which it is necessary to restore a balance between being too 'thick-skinned' and too 'thin-skinned'. We have already recommended it as a stimulant for the warmth organism, when it acts as a gateway for the forces of the warmth ether. The same applies to barley, only with more emphasis on the aspect of light.

The silica dynamics of the human organism can be strongly

stimulated by honey. In its six-sided combs, honey is impregnated by the forces of silica. Even the ancient Greek potters knew that the shape of a vessel influences whatever it contains. Thus in ancient days oil was preserved in specially-shaped jars. So honey, too, receives from its six-sided combs a unique formative impregnation related to silica. Thus as a food it takes with it into the human organism the same formative tendencies as those shown by silica when it forms six-sided crystals. Within the human organism, this tendency then first has to be overcome, because it is a principle imposed from without. Man's central component, his ego, is called upon to do this. The formative principles which, with the help of the silica organism, infuse all the tissues of the body take their cue from the human being's ego.

Honey is a valuable ingredient in a diet aimed at cancer prevention because to counteract cancer it is necessary to stimulate the dynamics of silica so that the cells multiplying formlessly may once again be contained properly by the principles of form. However, honey should be regarded as a medicine and administered in small doses only—not more than half a teaspoon twice daily.

Raw vegetables and salads, too, provide a strong stimulus for the silica processes in the human organism. Rudolf Steiner recommends that doctors prescribe potentized silica together with a diet of raw foods, for raw vegetables and salads awaken formative processes. Fruits, too, especially apples, are bearers of silica processes. So we see a variety of possibilities to work against cancer with the help of silica.

9. THE LIVER AS THE CHIELF ORGAN FOR METABOLISM AND DETOXIFICATION

The Liver and Cancer. Diet as a Preventative Measure

Claims are inevitably made on the liver both of cancer patients and of those with pre-cancerous conditions. Cancer is accompanied by disorders of the metabolism which of necessity have their impact on the chief metabolic organ. Added to this is the toxic state a tumour sets up in the organism. The main burden of breaking down and eliminating poisons rests with the liver, so that its capacity to function well has a considerable bearing on the outcome of the illness.

So in cancer prevention and cancer therapy it is essential to support the liver with a suitable diet. Rich dishes, such as anything fried in fat, are avoided. And since the liver is an intrinsic part of the warmth processes in the organism—the Russian word for it is connected with the word for 'to bake in an oven'—cold foods are unsuitable. Cold drinks should be warmed up to room temperature before consumption.

The liver also regulates the water balance and thus our thirst. To promote the function of detoxification and stimulate elimination patients should drink plenty. There are mineral waters which are particularly good for the liver. The circulation of liquid is also stimulated by setting aside from time to time a day during which only rice is eaten. Some herb teas, such as those containing St John's wort or yarrow, are also beneficial for the liver.

The liver produces glycogen, animal starch, from carbohydrates. Whole grains in the diet stimulate this function, but they must be finely ground and allowed sufficient time to swell. White flour and white beet sugar burden the carbohydrate metabolism because they lack essential elements. Fruits should be well ripened. In the evening, if liver function is weak, they are more easily digested when lightly stewed rather than raw. For the midday meal a tart apple or a grapefruit is more digestible before the meal rather than after. Dried fruits are usually well tolerated, especially apricots—but they must be unsulphured! Some of the vegetables eaten each day should be taken raw. Lactic-fermented vegetables are also easily digested.

Protein, too, is needed by the liver. The amounts required can usually be obtained from whole-grain foods, supplemented by dairy products such as soured milk and quark, of Demeter quality where possible (see Chapter 12). Only fresh products should be used. Unsuitable proteins easily lead to putrefaction in the intestines, which destroys the healthy intestinal flora. This burdens the liver. In this connection mention may be made of foci of infection such as bad teeth, tonsils or sinuses. In the interest of cancer prevention, with regard to liver function, these must definitely be treated.

Care should be taken with fats. Spread butter thinly on bread, use only the best culinary oils and add these only after cooking. Avoid anything fried.

Minerals and trace elements which are essential for liver metabolism are derived from vegetables and salads, and above all cereal grains.

Which grains are most suitable for the liver? Rye is rich in potassium, which is important for a healthy liver. Millet promotes warmth, as already mentioned, and oats contain valuable protein. Barley is good for the liver because of its carbohydrate content, which tends to be converted into sweet malt, and also its rich mineral content. Rice is good because its protein does not form the gluten layer enclosing the grain but is present throughout the inner part of the grain. Whole-grain wheat is also easily digested, as are buckwheat and maize (sweet-corn).

Culinary herbs are extremely valuable in all dishes, but especially in those based on cereal grains. Labiatae such as marjoram and basil have warmth properties and therefore benefit the liver. Umbelliferae such as caraway seeds, fennel, lovage relieve congestion in the airy organism and bring about a general sense of well-being. Among the spices of the Far East are many which benefit the liver. Ginger, turmeric and mace stimulate its activity.

Culinary herbs must be consciously tasted. If they are thoughtlessly swallowed they have no effect whatever.

This brings us to the important connection between the liver and the sense of taste. The liver, too, has a sense of taste. What we miss with our taste buds, or what we mistake for something else, is correctly perceived by the liver, which is not easily cheated. Indeed, it is easily offended. It reacts to all denatured foods laden with additives with a gesture of abhorrence, objecting to tastes which do not appeal to it. Thus it is forced to suffer for all the things we carelessly let through when we eat.

We do the liver a good turn if we taste everything thoroughly in our mouth, if we explore the food with our sense of taste. When we let our liver participate in this way we gradually build up a healthy instinct with regard to food.

Another thing which damages the liver is inattentive, hasty eating resulting from pressure of time. People in certain professions, for instance nurses, who are often forced to swallow their food in a great hurry, tend to suffer from liver disorders.

A bitter taste stimulates the liver, for instance that of chicory, green salads or spices such as ginger. A small cup of vegetable broth or bitter herb tea drunk at the start of a meal stimulates the liver.

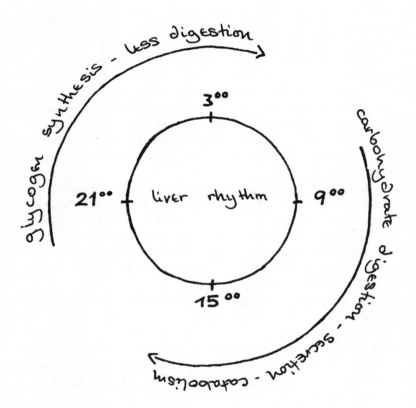

From time to time it is good for the liver if we take into account the alternating phases of its rhythm. There are two main functional phases which alternate regularly in accord with the path of the sun: a secretory phase in which the secretion of digestive juices dominates, and a phase in which glycogen is synthesized. The first phase reaches its peak at 3 o'clock in the afternoon, the second at 3 o'clock in the morning. Thus during the first part of the day we should give preference to foods which require the secretion of digestive juices, in other words we should eat well. As the saying goes: In the morning eat like a king, at midday like a nobleman and in the evening like a beggar. Well, we need not actually eat like a beggar in the evening. But as the liver begins to build up glycogen in the evening, we can offer it mainly carbohydrates and dishes more on the sweet side. By following this rhythm we support the liver. Anything fatty is to be treated with caution in the evening.

10. RHYTHMS

The alternating phases of the liver are a part of an overall pattern of rhythms. Together with other functions in the organism, such as temperature changes, blood sugar level and the diurnal variations in blood pressure, they are bound to the course of the sun. The earth itself also undergoes such phases. The barometer, for instance, has high and low points at 3 pm and 3 am, regardless of whether an area of high or low pressure happens to be passing. The field of electrical tension also participates in this alternation.

Other rhythms, too, work in the human organism. Our blood circulates in unison with the beating of our heart. The air organism moves in concert with our breathing. These rhythms are to a certain extent individual to each human being, yet they are linked to a wider cosmic order. Rudolf Steiner has pointed out that there is a hidden link between the human being's respiratory rhythm and the passage of the sun through the signs of Zodiac. On an average, 18 breaths are drawn every minute, or 25,920 every day. The sun takes exactly as many years to complete the circle of the Zodiac at the spring equinox.

When different functional cycles meet, they relate in a living way to reach a balance. In the mechanical world hard substances meet head-on, but in the human organism one rhythmic variation relates to another. Thus the rhythm of the abdomen relates to the rhythm of the blood circulation and this in turn is bound up with the rhythm of breathing in and out. This is then repeated right up to the system of nerves and senses in the head. For the column of the spinal fluid, which flows into the cerebral fluid, pulsates with the rhythm of respiration. It rises on the in-breath and falls on the out-breath. As it rises it flows into the cerebral sinuses where its waves break as though on a shore, and then it flows back as the water recedes. Thus the breathing rhythm is sensed in the head and everything is balanced out, far beneath the threshold of consciousness, naturally.

Thus between the polar opposites of the system of nerves and senses on the one hand and the metabolism on the other—neither of which is founded on a rhythm of its own—there exists in the chest a strong central rhythm represented by breathing and heart action.

This central rhythm is underlined by the fact that pulse and breathing are adjusted to one another. This is shown by the pulse-respiration ratio of 4:1, roughly four pulse beats to one breath. Certain disorders can lead to variations ranging from 8:1 to 3:1, and nutrition can influence this too.

Protein and iron have an interesting rhythmical relationship. In a way they may be seen to be antagonists. Protein serves the processes of life, growth and regeneration. It wells up and is the bearer of creative forces. Iron gives form to living substance and causes it to serve the development of consciousness. With the help of iron, substances are formed in the human organism which can become bearers of the self-conscious spirit. This formation of substances must not be allowed to fall under the influence of vital forces.

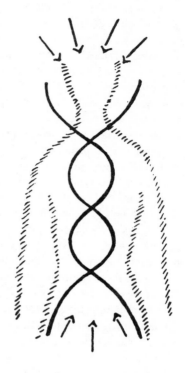

In human blood there is a certain ratio between protein and iron. Does this remain steady or can variations be observed? If so, what kind? Are they similar to the daily character of other rhythms?

Not surprisingly, in the morning the quota is tipped in favour of iron, whereas towards evening protein becomes more prominent. This gives expression to the fact that in the morning our organism is adjusted to activity; clarity and alertness of consciousness come with the new day. Then, as night approaches, organic regeneration sets in; our thoughts tend to lose their clear outline and become indeterminate.

Human beings are not at the mercy of these rhythms. They are free to dream in the morning if they like, and to think clearly in the evening.

But they might do both with more success if they choose the time appropriate to each.

The iron and protein balances are determined by a higher order of metabolism. In the blood stream, red blood corpuscles constantly disintegrate, freeing iron. This is first taken in by the liver in an assimilation phase and then given out again in a secretory phase serving either the formation of bile or the formation of blood in the bone marrow.

As we have seen, the liver has an assimilatory phase of glycogen synthesis and a phase in which bile is secreted. Both run parallel with the daily variations in iron levels.

In the case of protein the process is different. The liver does not absorb it at night and store it as it does glycogen. Instead in an organic process of synthesis it is newly formed in the serum during the evening and night. Thus the internal regenerative processes which serve life are initiated. As morning approaches, the organism is tuned more to the processes of digestion in stomach and intestines, that is the secretory phase in which protein is broken down. This is why it is preferable to eat protein meals before 3 pm.

How do these rhythmic principles work in the cancer patient? The fact alone that the cancer cell does not breathe expresses its exclusion from the rhythms of the organism in which it has no part. The actual formation of a tumour is preceded, however, by a slow process in which cells degenerate and increasingly enter a phase void of any rhythm. So in cancer prevention it is important to activate all the rhythmical processes. There is then a hope that the forces which operate on a higher level can succeed in retaining all cells within the totality, which is always based on rhythms. This can be tackled in various ways, but here we are concerned with the extent to which these processes can be influenced by nutrition.

The rhythmical processes in the human organism are best promoted by foods from plants which have been grown in accordance with the rhythms of the cosmos. If sowing, planting, tilling and harvesting can be done at the moment when the cosmic constellations are best for each particular fruit or vegetable, then the formative forces in the plants are woven in a healing and rhythmical way so that the produce has a nutritional quality which can stimulate corresponding rhythms in the human organism. Conversely, produce grown on soil treated with mineral fertilizers is so hard and coarse that it can no longer react to the influence of cosmic rhythms. Therefore it can in turn not stimulate the rhythmical processes in the human being in the degree that is possible for produce grown by the bio-dynamic method.[23]

The organ which first takes in the rhythms of the foods eaten and then leads them over into the individual rhythm of the human etheric body is the spleen. Ancient tradition placed the spleen under the influence of Saturn. Saturn's rings express its particular function. It creates a sphere around our solar system which acts as a barrier to influences from other starry worlds, thus enabling our solar system to unfold and maintain its own rhythm.

The spleen works in the same way in the human being. It is active chiefly in the etheric realm. For rhythm is a characteristic of life, a movement, a vibration, a kind of resounding which works from the etheric sphere into the visible world, giving it order and shape. Because the spleen is so very much an etheric organ it is possible for the physical organ to be removed without any detrimental consequences. Its function is continued by what is known as an 'accessory' spleen which is brought into being out of the etheric realm.

When food has been eaten, the spleen tackles the inner rhythm of the substances and causes it to conform to a certain extent to the individual rhythm of the blood system. In doing so, the spleen becomes enlarged and remains so for several hours.

The spleen also has the task of bringing balance into the imbalance brought about by irregular meals. Especially in children it is overtaxed by the bad habit of eating between meals and a person's whole rhythmical system can be damaged by this. In contrast, the spleen is strengthened when meals are taken regularly in a rhythmical way.

The transition, which is accomplished by the spleen, from the activity of digestion to the activity of circulation makes particular demands on the organism. Rudolf Steiner says in this connection:[24] 'What is the activity of digestion? It is metabolism tending towards something rhythmical, unfolding into something rhythmical. Digestive activity is metabolism which is taken up by the rhythm of the circulatory organs.' This takes place above all in the tissue fluids. This is where the actual nourishing takes place: 'It is wrong to suppose that it is merely the intake of foods which keeps human beings alive. What truly nourishes them is the living activity of the living interplay of forces in the tissue fluids.' And it is in the tissue fluids that we can seek the activity of the spleen.

In these processes an important part is played by the conscious attention paid to tasting what we eat. H. Glatzel[25] found that

43

unseasoned foods placed a strain on the heart because every pulse beat brought an increased amount of blood to it. This increased blood flow did not occur when foods were well-seasoned and consciously tasted.

The diaphragm brings about a living balance between the rhythms of the abdominal and thoracic cavities. It moves because we breathe and with this rhythm it touches the moving intestines. This can be used therapeutically for a gentle massage of the intestines which takes into account the movement of the diaphragm. Many people's breathing is quite shallow. Their diaphragm is either too relaxed or inclined to spasm, and thus the rhythm of the breathing fails to affect the intestines. The consequences are disorders of intestinal movement leading to insufficient absorption and persistent constipation.

The Four Seasons

The four seasons represent one of the larger rhythms. Nature changes during the course of the year and the human organism is adjusted to this rhythm of spring, summer, autumn and winter. This makes it necessary to adjust our food and in Europe we can do this in accordance with what nature gives us in each season. In addition some degree of balance can be achieved by means of storing and preserving foods.

Spring

The name of the month of February points to the health aspect of the spring, for it is derived from the Latin *febris*, meaning fever, cleansing. Ancient wisdom lies in this name: People are called to 'spring clean' their organism in good time. All the 'dust' and 'slag' that has been collected over the winter must be thrown out. Justice is also done in this respect by the old custom, which is not only religious, of fasting at this time of the year. There is no need to undertake this to any extreme. Protein and fat should be reduced. Meat-eaters can do without meat and also fish for a while. Instead there will be plenty of raw vegetables on the menu, perhaps exclusively on some days, accompanied by soured milk products. A good purifying dose of sulphur principles can be achieved with onions, garlic, horse radish, chives and radishes of all varieties.

When after a few weeks the first greenery starts to emerge from the soil we can enrich our meals with all sorts of good gifts of nature: nettles, dandelion leaves, ground elder, sorrel and many other herbs enliven metabolism and stimulate blood formation. But take care when gathering them. Avoid any spot which might have been sprayed, for this practice is unfortunately more widespread than one might expect.

Soon the young birch leaves start to sprout and a course of birch elixir does everyone good, especially the elderly. Blood-cleansing spring cures help the organism to make a fresh start. Formative processes such as that governed by silica should be stimulated. Cereal grains are especially suitable for this. After the cleansing process, milk products, especially from soured milk, are good for bringing about an upsurge of strength. Honey is beneficial all the year round.

Summer

In the summer all the greening and flowering reaches its peak. The earth breathes its soul right out and offers itself up to the cosmos. A principle is at work here which the alchemists called the 'sulphur principle'. They included in it everything which dissolves, which strives outwards towards the periphery, everything related to warmth and of a fiery nature. In sulphur we can see the earthly substance which most clearly embodies this principle. Whatever streams out in the flowering process, filling the earth with summer fragrance and aroma, whatever makes the colours so rich and luminous, whatever fills us with warmth and well-being, all such things are expressions of the sulphur principle.

Human beings, too, flow out into their environment in the summer. They enjoy giving themselves up to the summer heat and the shining quality of nature, for in them, also, the sulphur processes are at work. But they must not give themselves up entirely or they would become dreamers and lose their clarity of consciousness. Iron—the main constituent of human blood—helps to overcome excessive sulphur processes.

So what foods should we chose to eat during the summer? The sulphur processes, which are to some extent inherent in the human organism, need some support through nutrition in the metabolic area. Much that nature gives us in the summer is suitable for this, for everything is 'sulphurous' to some extent. However, onions and other heavily sulphurous spices should be used sparingly so that the sulphur processes do not become over-stimulated.

To prevent this by means of nutrition we can see to it that iron is eaten. One of the most important 'iron' plants is the nettle. It is quite in order to continue eating nettles right into the summer if they are blanched or gently boiled and improved by the addition of cream and spices such as nutmeg. They can also be mixed raw amongst other herbs. Cereal grains also stimulate iron metabolism. In the summer we give precedence to the more 'flowerlike' grains of millet, oats, rice, buckwheat and barley.

All kinds of fruit are very popular in the summer. They can be eaten with dairy products, especially soured milk which demands less sugar than fresh milk. If some sweetener is needed, refined sugar should be avoided, and honey, malt extract, syrup or fruit juice concentrates used instead.

Autumn

Autumn is the season of ripening and harvesting. As signs of gratitude to the divine creative powers, fruits, grains and all sorts of produce are laid before the altar in the churches. Whenever we eat we should join in this gesture of awe before the forces of life which give us our food.

The chief gift of the autumn are fruits. Apples, pears, plums, apricots, peaches, grapes and many others give us pleasure by their freshness and fragrance. Our organism needs this stimulus so that it can be armed when the cold of winter approaches. Of course we shall preserve some for the dark part of the year. Apart from proper storage, the best method is drying.

What do fruits do for the human organism when eaten? The whole of the metabolism is enlivened, and protein formation in the abdominal organs is especially stimulated. The actual substances of proteins and fats are present only in tiny amounts, but what works in the fruits is a living dynamic: the warmth of the sun which has united with them, and the aromatic sweetness which we owe to this warmth. When soil and plants are cultivated by the bio-dynamic method this develops to the full.

Nuts are another goodly gift of autumn. Hazelnuts nourish the nerves. It is a good idea to give children about seven hazelnuts every morning as part of their school snack.

The seeds of some plants, such as olive, safflower, sunflower, rape and linseed, yield high-quality oils which kindle the warmth processes in the human organism right through the autumn and into winter.

This brings us to the basic theme of nutrition at this time of the year: thorough warming through and stimulation of inner mobility. This is something we need to demand of our soul-life too, for is there not a threat of the coldness of the intellect spreading into every sphere, forcing warmth of heart to atrophy and the soul to be paralyzed?

Properly understood, nutrition is not something to be taken in isolation. It should be included among all the healing impulses in human life as a whole.

Winter

During the winter the earth takes all life back into itself as though breathing in. The forces which unfolded during spring and summer in the greening of the plants, which streamed outwards in the flowers, and brought about the ripening of the seeds in the autumn, have now returned to the womb of the earth. But the soil is very much alive, particularly where the metabolism of minerals is concerned. Returning once more to the medieval alchemists, we can now speak of salt processes. The plant world inside the earth plays a lively part in these, for instance winter cereals. Rye sends its roots down to a depth of one and a half metres. There it is always warm and the world of microorganisms immensely lively, even when there is a biting frost on the surface.

And what about human beings? Plant roots with their mineral forces are related to the human head. For the head is the most solid, most mineralized part of the body. Thought processes, too, are supported by salt processes in the brain. Thinking is easiest in the winter, and the senses are bright and clear. Many animals hibernate, but human beings are especially called upon by what is going on in nature to be awake and, in self-knowledge and self-responsibility, to form judgements based on spiritual insights.

Cereal grains, our staple food, support these processes because of their relationship to light and their very definite mineral quality. The same can be said of root vegetables which are available in many variations. Other vegetables too, such as salads and fruits which are harvested in winter or have been stored in the autumn, complete our menu. They participate in the winter processes to which the human organism is now attuned. This also applies to winter apples. Welcome additions to our winter menu come in the form of preserved summer and autumn produce, especially lactic-fermented vegetables and dried fruits, as well as honey. Bio-dynamic oranges are an occasional delicacy. However, as a general rule the nature of the winter season should be taken into account. Thus such things as frozen strawberries are questionable. Our healthy instinct will help us to choose our foods to suit the season.

All these things are very important for the cancer patient and also with regard to cancer prevention. The rhythmical processes embrace the forces needed to help all the different organs find their proper place in the total order of the body once again.

47

11. CEREAL GRAINS IN THE DIET OF CANCER PATIENTS

In much of the world, cereal grains are one of the staple foods, so what part do they play in cancer prevention and in the diet of cancer patients? Are they able to stimulate forces which can counteract a process in which tissues are overcome by the heaviness of physical substance and in danger of falling away from the influence of the etheric creative forces? (See Chapter 2.)

How do grains ripen? In the early stage they are still soft and juicy or 'milky' and contain few mineral substances. Then in the heat of the summer sun the process is rounded off. The substance of the seeds dries out. Starch, proteins and fats solidify and minerals such as calcium, phosphorus, magnesium and silica are deposited. The mineralizing, solidifying forces seem to gain the upper hand, making the seeds look almost as if they were dead.

But they are not. Far from it, for cereal grains become an incomparable foodstuff because the etheric creative forces have entered so strongly with the sun's rays into the world of physical substance that they are now able to take hold of the mineralizing process and prevent this substance from sinking down entirely into the world of gravity. The way in which they germinate demonstrates how very much alive cereal grains are. Here the solidified mineral substances are loosened and dissolved as life begins to rise up again. Grains buried 4,000 years ago in Egyptian pyramids have been successfully brought to germination. What a demonstration of the dynamic forces of life resting in them! This achievement on the part of the plant is based on a process which can help to overcome a disposition to cancer. Gravity is overcome and substances are once more taken up by the forces of dynamic life.

However, this effect of cereal grain foods cannot be taken for granted today. Modern methods of seed breeding, of cultivation with massive applications of mineral fertilizers, and above all the over-refining of flour all lead to a considerable decrease in quality. Ordinary production methods cause the loss of 70-85% of minerals, 40-90%

of trace elements, 65-85% of water-soluble vitamins, and 70-85% of roughage. B. Thomas[26] writes: 'With regard to breeding, fertilizers, machines for milling and baking, and the manufacture of various production aids, large-scale mass production is financially geared for years to come to the production of endosperm products, i.e. white flour.'

Our choice of cereals with regard to cancer will vary from case to case, depending on the constitution of the individuals concerned, the state of their digestive system and the severity of their illness.

Rye shows a high degree of mineralization, demonstrated by its strong root formation, the height of its stems and the size of its ears. It is rich in silica, which shows its relationship to light, as does its capacity to be grown at high altitudes. Rye-based foods give us formative forces and activate our light metabolism. Its potassium content means that it has a favourable effect on the liver.

Barley is also strong in silica processes and thus related to light. It stimulates the function of nerves and sense organs and promotes faculties of concentration. Sugar processes are strong in barleycorns, as is shown by their suitability for malting. The outer layers are rich in Vitamin B_1, which can stimulate sugar metabolism in the cells. To increase this nutritional effect, the barley should be slow dried (see *Slow Drying* in Chapter 12) before coarse grinding. In some European countries is is available in health shops under the name of *Demeter 'Thermo'-Getreide* (Demeter thermally treated grain).

Oats are a cereal belonging to Europe's northern regions, where they flourish best in the cool, damp climate of the coast. Here they develop a hidden fire process which is revealed in their high fat content and which makes those who eat them lively. Oats thus go with the choleric temperament. In the diet, oats are not so much a stimulus for the system of nerves and senses, that is the conscious pole of the human being, but rather for the system of metabolism and limbs, for their effect is one of warming through and stimulating activity. Thus they are also a help for people suffering from lack of initiative and drive.

The carbohydrates in oats require less insulin to break them down. In addition oats stimulate insulin production by the pancreas, thus acting in a genuinely healing way with regard to diabetes. This effect can also be useful in the case of cancer.

For dietary purposes it is useful to slow dry oats (see Chapter 12) and then grind them finely. Whether sweet or savoury, the resulting dish is tasty and easily digested. To relieve the burden on the metabolism a number of 'oat days' are recommended.

Millet with its loose, effervescent panicle and tiny mobile grains reveals both its own nature and how it works on the human being. It bears the stamp of silica and as a food it supports the functions of skin and sense organs. It also stimulates warmth processes. The latter quality, and also its relationship to silica, makes it one of the main ingredients in a diet aimed at preventing cancer (see Chapter 8).

A diet which includes millet can be a help in connection with one of the causes of cancer, namely the over-stimulation of all the senses in modern life (see Chapter 3). To boost the effect of diets using raw vegetables and salads it is recommended that some cooked millet be included (see Chapter 12).

Rice is closely related to the element of water. Paddy fields have to be flooded so that the water can wash around the young rice plants. The grains are highly nutritious and very easily digested. For diet purposes it is used because of its capacity to promote elimination and stimulate flow in the fluid organism.

Maize (sweet corn) is important in dietetics because it contains no gluten. Maize flour cannot be baked into bread, but all maize products are extremely valuable in diets for those who are allergic to the protein in cereal grains.

Most traditional maize dishes are strongly seasoned. This is to redeem the maize from its earthy heaviness which it shows in its huge growth and massive cobs which develop in the leafy region of the plant. Maize is also rich in carotene and we can gain much pleasure from the golden colour of all maize dishes.

Wheat among all the cereal grains stands harmoniously in the middle. It is easily digested and nourishes all the organs equally. Together with rye it is the main bread cereal. It is favoured by many for diets using sprouted seeds and live grain mueslis.

All cereals can be combined in many ways with vegetables, salads, fruits and dairy products. To complete their effect they need to be well seasoned with herbs, and it is a good idea to add some fine oil after cooking.

12. PRACTICAL GUIDELINES

From what has been said in the foregoing chapters it can be seen that there are indeed fundamental guidelines both for the diet of cancer patients and for nutrition in the service of general cancer prevention. A number of practical suggestions have already been made which will now be added to and summarized.

Cultivation and Processing of Plant Products

Whenever possible, use produce grown by the bio-dynamic method, but if this is not available, organically grown produce will have to suffice. Anything grown with mineral fertilizers or treated with chemical sprays is to be avoided. This also applies to produce treated with chemicals to keep it fresh, to preserve it, to prevent mould or improve appearance or flavour. In some countries it is not easy to keep to these rules, but almost everywhere now it is possible, by dint of sufficient enquiries, to find sources of unspoilt foods. Cancer is serious enough to warrant every effort. (For addresses in English-speaking countries, see list at the end of the Bibliography.)

Let us now turn to the practical application of the different foods.

Cereal Grains

There are a number of books on the preparing and cooking of grain dishes,[27,28] but here are a few general rules. For ordinary dishes grains can be used whole or freshly ground. They should be 'developed' by prior soaking (3-10 hours), after which they are cooked over a very gentle heat and then left to stand while they absorb the rest of the liquid. For eating raw in the form of muesli there are flakes which have already been subjected to a warmth process. Grains may also be slow dried before grinding, after which they only need to be soaked before using. Slow drying is equivalent to the final ripening in the ear after cutting (stooks). Sick people should be given raw grains only with the doctor's permission.

Slow drying: The grains are moistened, spread thinly on a baking tray and left in the oven for one hour at a temperature of about

70°C. They give off a pleasant, tangy aroma and they should not be allowed to go brown. Treated like this, even oats can easily be ground without gumming up the grinder because of their high fat content. On the continent of Europe slow dried grain is available under the brand name of *'Thermo'-Getreide*.

Sprouted grains: Equipment for sprouting grains is now available on the market. The basic method without special equipment is as follows: A thin layer of grains is placed in a large bowl with twice their amount of water and left to stand for 36 hours at a temperature of below 15°. The grains swell by absorbing all the water. Then they are laid not more than two grains deep on muslin stretched over a frame. At a temperature of about 17° they are left to sprout for 3 days. To keep them moist spray at intervals.

Sprouted grains are eaten raw. Honey, nuts, soured milk, grated apple or freshly chopped herbs can be added to taste.

Bread: Of all foods, bread is the most suitable for human beings. It is extremely worrying that the quality of this most fundamental of foods should have become so downgraded by today's production methods. Quite apart from the quality of the seed grains, and the methods of cultivation and storage, current methods of milling with steel rollers and the making of white flour lead to a considerable decrease in quality.

In the baking process synthetic acids and compressed yeast are used. This is a very questionable method which shortens the laborious sour dough process but fails to 'develop' the grain sufficiently. The bread is then further devalued by the use of chemicals which prevent mould.[29]

For cancer patients and cancer prevention high-quality bread is a must. When available, bread of the 'Demeter' standard is best, since it guarantees not only the special care of the grain itself, starting with its cultivation, but also the use of baking methods which fully 'develop' the freshly milled grain.

Many people who are concerned about what they eat bake their own bread.[29] For bread it is good to mix the four cereals indigenous to Europe: wheat, rye, barley and oats. But for other foods it is best to use one type of grain at a time, since each requires a different method of preparation which brings out its own essential nature which it is good to experience when it is eaten.

Herbs and Spices

Herbs and spices are bearers of light and warmth and therefore a valuable part of a cancer diet. By forming essential oils, resins and aromatic substances they have taken the flowering process into other parts of the plant such as the leaves, stems, roots or seeds. They complement cereal grains, which have little aroma of their own. They also stimulate the digestive processes if they are tasted attentively.

Milk and Dairy Products

As far as cancer is concerned, it is better to do without commercially produced milk and turn to **soured milk products** instead.

Plain **buttermilk** is an ideal drink. As a by-product of butter making it contains only 0.1-0.3% fat but almost all the mineral salts and all the milk proteins. **Kefir** is a soured milk with an effervescent taste. It is produced by kefir grains which consist, amongst other things, of yeast moulds. These produce small amounts of carbon dioxide and alcohol amounting to 0.2-1%, which can give cause for concern!

Live yogurt is produced with the help of special lactic acid bacteria, especially *Lactobacillus acidophilus* which occurs in the human gut.

Quark, or the French version **Fromage Frais**, is a versatile soured milk product. If possible buy Demeter quark, since the ordinary products usually have fewer living qualities because they are mechanically thickened. Better still, make it at home. Suspend sour milk in a muslin bag till all the whey has run out. The **whey** can be used for baking bread. **Cheese** should also be of Demeter quality were possible, and all processed cheeses should be avoided because they contain phosphates. Matured cheeses which are free of nitrates are preferred.

Vegetables

In order to use the different vegetables in a meaningful way for dietary purposes, we have to make the threefold plant our starting point and distinguish between:

1. Roots and tubers
2. Leaves and stems
3. Flowers and fruits.

The first group includes carrots, swedes, parsnips, salsify, beetroot, celeriac, radish and Teltow turnips. Jerusalem artichokes and potatoes are tubers. As discussed elsewhere, potatoes are to be avoided in a cancer diet.

The second group includes the leaf vegetables spinach, various types of cabbage, fennel and lettuce and the stem vegetables chicory, leek, asparagus, Swiss chard and kohlrabi.

In the third group we have flower vegetables such as cauliflower, Brussels sprouts, broccoli, globe artichokes as well as immature pods such as garden peas, mangetout and French and runner beans. Among the fruits are pumpkin, cucumbers, courgettes and melons.

Tomatoes are not suitable in a cancer diet. Green peppers and aubergines are also plants of the deadly nightshade family and should be used sparingly. Among the pulses, haricot beans, lentils and unfermented soyabeans should be avoided because of their massive protein processes.

Fungi (mushrooms) are not suitable for human consumption. Their lightless, hasty growth soon ends in toxic decomposition and is reminiscent of the growth of a tumour.

The three parts of the plant each unfold different qualities and stand in different relationships to their environment. The flower together with the fruit and seed formation develops the strongest metabolic activity and is the warmest part of the plant. The root, in contrast, unites with the dark, moist and cool soil and comes to grips with the mineral element. Leaf and stem mediate between these two polar opposites of above and below. In them the plant breathes and its sap circulates.

Similar functional areas may be distinguished in the human being. In the chest lies the middle sphere which breathes and which contains the central organ of the circulation of fluids. Thus the middle, rhythmic region in man corresponds to the leaf and stem region in the plant. In the head consciousness unfolds, supported by fine salt and mineral processes; to think properly we have to keep a cool head. So here we are reminded of the root region of the plant. And finally our metabolic system with its warmth activity points to the flower and fruit of the plant.

Thoughts such as this are not idle allegorical fancies but a challenge to us to use them in practice as a foundation for nutrition. With root vegetables, processes in the region of nerves and senses can be stimulated; leaf and stem vegetables help to activate heart and lungs; and flower, fruit and seed vegetables stimulate the building up and functioning of the metabolic organs.

Of course we stop short of building up a rigid scheme to which we have to adhere at all costs. Often various principles join forces and work together. Thus though the carrot is a typical root vegetable, its orange colour and sweet taste are characteristic of a fruit. We might call it a 'root fruit'.

In normal nutrition we endeavour to include all parts of the threefold plant in our diet. Thus a root vegetable can be complemented by parsley representing the leaf element, honey representing the flower, and fennel or caraway or mustard seeds, or oil, representing the seed principle.

For a cancer diet, however, our starting point is the consideration of which function we want to address. Whatever else we do, though, we must strengthen the rhythmical middle region. Then, to work against too great a rigidity fruits and flowers are given preference, while to strengthen the formative forces more emphasis is laid on vegetables of the root variety. And in every recommendation the constitution of the patient is taken into account.

Lactic-fermented Produce

Lactic-fermented vegetables: As mentioned earlier, these have a healing effect where cancer is concerned. They are obtainable in good health food stores under the 'Eden' trademark, and can also be prepared at home. For those who read German Frau Annelies Schöneck's book *Milchsaure Gärung* (Lactic Fermentation)[30] can be recommended.

Lactic-fermented Bread Drink: This beverage, invented by Wilhelm Kanne,[31] is a valuable aid in conjunction with cancer therapy and also as a preventative measure. It is a refreshing, strengthening drink which can be sweetened with honey or combined with herb teas or mineral water. It may be warmed by standing the jug or mug in a pan of hot water. It is sometimes available in health food shops. A similar drink, kvass, can be made at home.[32]

Fruits

Fruits are not very nutritious but they stimulate metabolic processes in the organism. Their function is dynamic in that they activate renewal processes and also counteract excessive acid levels in the tissues. Among the trace elements they contain, iron and silica may be emphasized.

The quality of fruits is extremely important. Disastrous abuses are committed by the use of chemicals in fruit cultivation. Also as a result of fertilizers which speed up growth, soft fruits keep less well and since the distance between producer and consumer is usually great, they are often harvested whilst still unripe and allowed to ripen in transit. As a result, sweetness and flavour fail to develop to the full.

Generally fruits are eaten raw but this need not become a strict rule. Many fruits, for instance bilberries (blueberries) gain in aroma and are made more digestible by gentle stewing.

Drying often brings out flavour and sweetness even more strongly. This is the case with apricots, figs and dates. Drying is indeed one of the best means of preserving fruits, and this goes for plums, apple slices, pears and bilberries. Before eating they must always be soaked, preferably over night.

Black currants, cherries, red grapes and bilberries are recommended because of their high content of respiratory enzymes, magnesium and iron. Hazelnuts are much appreciated if they are not too old. Peanuts and peanut oil are undesirable because of their uric acid content.

Fats

Fats are important for the organism's warmth production and also for cell respiration. Attention must therefore be paid to them with regard to cancer. (See Chapter 7).

The fats used must be those which kindle warmth processes without clogging up the warmth organism with 'cinders'. These are linseed oil, safflower oil, wheat germ oil, sunflower oil and Demeter rape oil.

The way the oil is extracted is important as regards its quality. It should be cold pressed and not chemically extracted, and we should chose the first pressing and check on the date. Linseed oil, in particular, turns rancid after quite a short while. Butter is the best fat for spreading on bread, so long as it is of the highest quality. The daily fat requirement varies from one individual to the next, but 40-60g (which includes hidden fats and cooking fats) may serve as a guideline.

Green lettuce in considerable amounts serves to stimulate the fat metabolism in human beings. According to Rudolf Steiner, the leaf is the original fat producer. We need only think of the fine fatty film which forms on the surface of lettuce leaves or even cabbage leaves. The nourishing factor in lettuce is a dynamic process in the formative forces which is stimulated by the minute amounts of fat in the green leaves.

Sugar

As stated in Chapter 5, white or brown beet sugar is not advantageous for the cancer patient and should also be avoided in a preventative diet. Sweetness in itself, however, if left in its natural state can be necessary and beneficial. There are many excellent products which may be used as sweeteners: pear or date juice concentrates, sugar beet or maple syrup, concentrated and crystallized juice of the sugar cane (succanate), honey, dried fruits. Ripe fruits are often so sweet that they require no additional sweetening. Many people, however, have become accustomed to excessive sweetness and lost their true sense of taste. As we know, this is a genuine addiction[33] which might need a planned withdrawal. This can best be achieved on the basis of whole grain foods. Synthetic sweeteners must be strictly avoided. Fructose is also a synthetic product extracted by electrolysis and has nothing in common with a natural fruit and its creative forces.

Honey

Honey is a unique food. Consider how it is prepared by the bees. They collect the delicious nectar from the flowers and mix it in their bodies with their own enzymes which are related to their stings. This gives the honey a unique quality which raises it to the level of a universal medicine. The honey in the beehive is kept at a constant temperature of 37°C, the same as that of human blood, while it matures in the combs. The combs are six-sided, like rock crystals. This is imprinted on the honey (see Chapter 8). In the six-sided combs it gains the formative forces of silica and is therefore highly prized as part of a cancer diet. As it is a medicine, not more than 1-2 teaspoons a day should be taken. Honey from flowers is preferable to that from pine woods because light has had a more intense effect on it.

Meat

As stated earlier, meat has no place in a cancer diet because protein should be taken only sparingly. In addition meat makes metabolism sluggish, which makes it easier for parts to fall away from the formative forces. The heaviness that is part of physical nature is dominant in cancer and the patient should therefore avoid all foods which place this kind of burden on the organism.

Another factor is the highly questionable quality of meat these days. Most meat on the market comes from intensively reared stock and the animals are all degenerate in some way and habituated to medication. Another consideration which ought to concern those occupied with the problem of cancer is that of the waste involved in rearing stock. Enormous amounts of grain are fed to cattle while hundreds of thousands of people die of hunger. If the industrialized countries were to halve their meat consumption, enough grain would be freed to cover the food deficit in the developing countries.

The many substances fed to stock or injected as medication lead to changes in the meat that are foreign to the species. All sorts of indefinable consequences, also with regard to cancer, take place in the human organism when such meat is eaten. Those who cannot do without meat should at least restrict themselves to products of Demeter quality. These are also available as meat preserves.

Beverages

Cancer patients should have plenty to drink every day so that the toxic substances resulting from tissue disintegration are washed away. Small amounts at a time should be drunk, rather than large amounts all at once. Healthy people, too, should stimulate their fluid organism. Suitable beverages are: the liquid in which barley, oats or linseed have been boiled; buttermilk or whey; vegetable broths; fruit juices (do not use refined sugar for sweetening); lactic-fermented vegetable juices. Very much to be recommended is Kanne's lactic-fermented Bread Drink. Various herb teas also have a good effect.

High Fibre Diet

Many cancer experts are of the opinion that one of the chief causes of cancer are the refined foods lacking in fibre (eg white flour) which are nowadays preferred in western countries. This is borne out by Burkitt's large-scale epidemiological studies (see Chapter 2) which show that a lack of fibre in the diet causes the intestinal processes to slow down. Presumably a delay in voiding waste causes damage to the intestinal flora and this leads to toxic effects which favour the growth of tumours. Populations with slower digestive processes were found to be more prone to cancer.

Whole grains contain the ideal fibre for stimulating intestinal motility. This is what is known as hemicellulose. It swells to form a soft mass, acts as a mild stimulant to the walls of the intestines and also binds intestinal toxins and acids.

In any cancerous condition regular bowel movements are essential and can be aided by taking bran, linseed, prunes, or Kanne's Bread Drink.

Raw Food Diet

Raw foods stimulate metabolic processes in the periphery of the organism. Silica processes are set in motion and formative forces brought to life. More energy is needed to digest raw foods but more energy is created as a result. However, we must be sure that the organism is capable of the initial exertion, so sick people should only be given a raw diet under the supervision of a doctor. If excessive demands are made on the capacity of the metabolism, this can have a weakening effect because emphasizing the processes in the periphery can deplete the inner constructive processes.

Raw food diets have proved efficacious for skin diseases, diabetes, rheumatism, gout, high blood pressure and weaknesses of the sense organs. Experience varies as far as cancer is concerned, no doubt because there are so many aspects to be taken into account with this disease, which befalls people of every constitution and can affect all the different organic systems. Time and again, however, raw food diets have brought about improvements in cancers.

Rudolf Breuss's Vegetable Juice Cure[34]

Definite successes have also been achieved by fasting combined with the drinking of vegetable juices (pressed) and certain herb teas. These cures have been developed by Rudolf Breuss, a health practitioner. He recommends daily consumption of the juice of 300 g beetroot, 100 g carrots, 100 g celeriac and 30 g radish, with the possible addition of one potato the size of a hen's egg. The addition of the potato poses a problem for us, since we stated in Chapter 4 that potatoes should be avoided altogether in connection with cancer. Breuss leaves us free to choose and recommends that patients should endeavour to use their instinct to sense whether the potato juice is advantageous or not.

All the vegetables are expressed in a juicer and then put through a fine sieve or muslin to eliminate a sediment which apart from tasting nasty can be 'food for the cancer'. The cure takes 42 days. Apart from sage tea, kidney tea (a mixture of equisetum, nettles, knotgrass and St John's wort) is drunk for three weeks of this period. Breuss also sets great store by herb robert tea. (Teas should be bought ready-mixed. Some of the herbs are poisonous and must only be used in the right proportions. Tr.)

The juices are sipped at frequent intervals in conjunction with the teas. Both must be thoroughly mixed with saliva before swallowing.

The Importance of Regular Mealtimes
Cancer patients often suffer from weakeness of the digestive glands and it is therefore recommended that they should take small meals at short intervals, usually once every two hours. However, in severe cases a tablespoonful can be given every quarter of an hour. As the patient improves, there can be a transition to intervals of half an hour, then an hour and finally two hours.

Zabel[5] mentions an Austrian physician, Salzborn, who obtained astonishing successes with this method. Above all a rhythmical regularity is necessary.

As already mentioned, it is good to take the liver rhythm into account by giving light, carbohydrate-rich meals in the evening and favouring fats and proteins in the morning and at midday.

And finally one more mention of a very important rule: Even the smallest amounts of food must be thoroughly chewed and mixed with saliva and also consciously tasted!

Suggestion for a Daily Menu Aimed at Cancer Prevention

Breakfast
1. Muesli made from grain flakes with honey, nuts, apples (fruit in season), soured milk. Or
2. Porridge with the same ingredients. Or
3. Freshly-ground grains soaked over night, cooked in the same water and left to absorb the moisture. Add the same ingredients as in 1. Or
4. Wholegrain bread, butter with quark or cheese or (if sweetness is craved) fruit concentrates or honey. An apple or fruit in season. Beverage: herb tea. Or
5. Quark mixed with linseed oil on crispbread, wholemeal rusks or crispy flakes.

Lunch

1. Cup of vegetable broth or bitter tea or, heated by standing the mug in warm water, lactic-fermented vegetable juice or Kanne Bread Drink.
2. Raw vegetables or salad.
3. Cereal grains—various dishes and rhythmical alternation of different kinds (see recipes[27,28]). Vegetables cooked or raw to go with the grains. Sauce made with herbs. If desired and suitable, various milk puddings, quark dessert or stewed fruit.

Evening Meal

1. Soup made with freshly ground grains and either herbs or stewed dried fruits.
2. Soured milk products.
3. Bread, butter, light cheeses, herb tea.

Between meals: herb teas, crispbread, wholemeal biscuits, fruit, nuts, honey, fruit juices, soured milk products, Kanne Bread Drink.

CONCLUSION

Cancer is a disease of our time caused by many unhealthy factors in present-day life. Those who contract it take upon themselves a part of the destiny of all mankind. Those who overcome it unite with the healing forces of the universe which lie behind all things and are available.

To have cancer can mean to take on a noble task, to accept a sacrifice that must be tackled by the individual concerned. Each will find his own way. For many, healing is possible, while others face a destiny of long suffering leading to death. But even here healing can be brought about at a higher level by inner conquest.

Proper nutrition helps patients to set free those forces out of which the higher ego can intervene in a healing way. This always calls for a holistic therapy which takes into account above all the patients' state of spirit and soul. This in the final analysis will determine the degree of physical healing which can take place. Therefore an attitude to nutrition which takes the spiritual aspects into account is vital for recovery. Medicines such as the mistletoe preparations and the tried and tested measures of naturopathy can activate all the healing forces at the patient's disposal, even when an operation is unavoidable.

This book is also intended as an encouragement to work against cancer in general. Nowadays even 'normal' nutrition needs to be therapeutic, since almost every individual harbours a dormant tendency towards this disease.

BIBLIOGRAPHY AND ADDRESSES

Although most of the books listed in this bibliography are available in German only, they are included here in the hope that they will be of assistance to some readers.

1. Rudolf Steiner *The Spiritual-Scientific Aspect of Therapy*, 9 lectures to doctors and medical students, 11-18 April 1921, (English text available in typescript only).

2. Dietrich Boie *Der Geistige Ursprung des Karzinoms* (The Spiritual Origin of Cancer) in *Die Drei*, Verlag Freies Geistesleben, Stuttgart November 1976.

3. Rudolf Steiner *Spiritual Science and Medicine*, Rudolf Steiner Publishing Company, London 1948, 20 lectures to doctors and medical students, 21 March-9 April 1921.

4. P. Schwarz in *Deutsches Ärzteblatt* 1970.

5. Werner Zabel *Die interne Krebstherapie und die Ernährung des Krebskranken* (Cancer Therapy and Nutrition for the Cancer Patient), Bircher-Benner Verlag, Bad Homburg.

6. D. G. Burkitt, J. Waldenström *Schnellere Darmpassage bei Naturkost* (Digestion Speeded Up by Natural Foods), Frankfurt 1972.

7. *Ernährungsrundbrief*, Booklet 36, published by the Arbeitskreis für Ernährungsforschung, Zwerweg 19, D-7263 Bad Liebenzell-Unterlengenhardt, German Federal Republic.

8. *Beiträge der biologisch-dynamischen Landwirtschaftsmethode in der Schweiz*, August 1982, Stockborn, Switzerland.

9. Gerhard Schmidt *Dynamische Ernährungslehre* (Dynamic Nutrition), Volume II, p.188-194, Proteus Verlag, St Gallen 1979.

10. Rudolf Steiner *Agriculture*, Bio-Dynamic Agricultural Association, London 1977, 8 lectures, 7—16 June 1924.

11. Rudolf Steiner *Cosmic Workings in Earth and Man*, lecture of 22 September 1923, Rudolf Steiner Publishing Company, London 1952

12. Gerhardt Schmidt in *Mitteilungen aus der Behandlung maligner Tumoren mit Viscum album*, Special Number 3-1970, Verein für Krebsforschung, Arlesheim, Switzerland.

13. Rudolf Steiner *Physiologisch-Therapeutisches auf Grundlage der Geisteswissenschaft*, lectures given in Dornach in March and April 1924.

14. J. Kuhl *Eine erfolgreiche Arznei-und Ernährungsbehandlung gutartiger und bösartiger Geschwulste* (Successful Treatment of Benign and Malignant Tumours with Medicaments and Nutrition) , Humata Verlag, Freiburg 1962.

15. Otto Wolff *Die Milchsäure in Wachstum und Gestaltung* (Lactic Acid in Growth and Formation) in *Mitteilungsblatt des Vereins für Krebsforschung*, Booklet VII,VIII, Arlesheim, February 1955.

16. Rudolf Steiner, lecture given on 6 January 1924.

17. Jacques Lusseyran *And There Was Light*, London 1964.

18. Herbert Sieweke *Anthroposophische Medizin* (Anthroposophical Medicine), Dornach 1959, Chapter 14.

19. Klara Zupic *Der Krebs als Lichtstoffwechselstörung* (Cancer as a Disorder of Light Metabolism), Verein für Krebsforschung, Arlesheim 1979.

20. R. Teubner, M. Rattermeyer and W. Mehlhardt *Neue Methode zur Feststellung der Qualität von Lebensmitteln* (New Method

for Determining the Quality of Foodstuffs) in *Ärztezeitschrift für Naturheilverfahren* 4.81.

21. Gerhard Schmidt *Zur Frage der Kältekonservierung von Lebensmitteln* (On the Question of Food Preservation by Freezing) in *Ernährungsrundbrief*, Booklets 35 and 36. (See Note 7)

22. Almar von Wistinghausen *Kiesel im Haushalt der Natur und in der Landwirtschaft* (Silica in Nature and in Agriculture) in *Ernährungsrundbrief*, Booklet 42. (See Note 7)

23. Maria Thun and Hans Heinze *Anbauversuche über Zusammenhänge zwischen Mondstellungen im Tierkreis und Kulturpflanzen* (Experiments to Determine Links between the Position of the Moon in the Zodiac and the Growth of Crops) in the series *Lebendige Erde*, Darmstadt 1973.

24. Rudolf Steiner *Curative Eurythmy* (English text available in typescript only).

25. H. Glatzel *Die Gewürze* (Herbs), Herford 1968.

26. B. Thomas *Nährstoffverluste bei der modernen Brotherstellung* (Loss of Nutrients in Modern Bread Production) in *Diaita in Erfahrungsheilkunde*, Heidelberg 1980/84.

27. Udo Renzenbrink *Zeitgemässe Getreide-Ernährung* (Cereal Grains in Contemporary Nutrition), Rudolf Geering Verlag, Dornach 1979.

28. Recipe booklet *Die Zubereitung von Getreide* (Grain Recipes), published by Arbeitskreis für Ernährungsforschung, 1982. (See Note 7)

29. Ada Pokorny *Die Verarbeitung des Getreides zu Brot und Gebäck*, (Grain in Bread, Cakes and Pastries) published by Arbeitskreis für Ernährungsforschung, 1980. (See Note 7)

30. Annelies Schöneck *Milchsaure Gärung zuhause* (Lactic Fermenting at Home), Karlsruhe 1979. (Bersgatan 10b, S-15020 Järna, Sweden).

31. Wilhelm Kanne Bakery, D-4670 Lünen/Westphalia, Im Geistwinkel 40, German Federal Republic.

32. To make Kvass see *Ernährungsrundbrief*, Booklet 40. (See Note 7)

33. Olaf Koob *Droge und Suchtentstehung* (Drugs and Dependence), leaflet published by Verein für ein erweitertes Heilwesen e.V., D-7263 Bad Liebenzell/Unterlengenhardt, German Federal Republic.

34. Rudolf Breuss *Krebs* (Cancer), obtainable from Versandbuchhandlung Margreiter, Im Hag 23, A-6714 Nüziders, or Hans Schmid, Gehrenberg 39, D-7988 Wangen/Allgäu.

Addresses for information on availability of bio-dynamic produce:

Bio-Dynamic Agricultural Association
Woodman Lane, Clent, Stourbridge,
West Midlands, DY9 9PX, UK

Bio-Dynamic Information Centre
Kawana, Boundary Street, Roseville,
NSW 2069, Australia

Bio-Dynamic Farming and Gardening Association
PO Box 425, Napier,
New Zealand

Bio-Dynamic Farming and Gardening Association Inc
PO Box 550, Kimberton,
PA 19442, USA

Society for Bio-Dynamic Farming and Gardening in Ontario
8 Cheval Court, Richmond Hill,
Ontario L4E 1H5, Canada

For the UK the following book marks shops which sell Bio-Dynamic produce with the Demeter and Biodyn Symbols: Alan Gear *The New Organic Food Guide*, J M Dent & Sons Ltd, London 1988, ISBN 0-460-02454-X.